THE No-Diet

Obesity Solution for Kids

Miriam B. Vos, MD, MSPH

The No-Diet Obesity Solution for Kids

Disclaimer

This publication provides accurate information on the subject matter covered. The publisher is not providing legal, medical, or other professional services. Reference herein to any specific commercial products, procedures, or services by trade name, trademark, manufacturer, or otherwise does not constitute or imply endorsement, recommendation, or favored status by the AGA Institute. The views and opinions of the author(s) expressed in this publication do not necessarily state or reflect those of the AGA Institute, and they shall not be used to advertise or endorse a product.

Printed in the United States of America

12 11 10 09   1 2 3 4 5 6

ISBN 978-1-60356-004-7

Library of Congress Control Number: 2009920609

For additional copies or information on licensing or translating this content, please contact:

4930 Del Ray Avenue
Bethesda, MD 20814-2513
www.gastro.org/publications
www.thenodietobesitysolutionforkids.com

To all of my patients and their families

Because each of you moves forward bravely,
despite the challenges

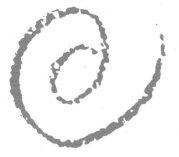

About the American Gastroenterological Association

The American Gastroenterological Association is the field's leading medical society and represents more than 17,000 members worldwide involved in all facets of gastroenterology practice, research, and education. The AGA Institute Press published *The No-Diet Obesity Solution for Kids* to support the health of our children and fight obesity as part of an association-wide obesity initiative.

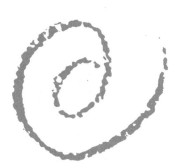

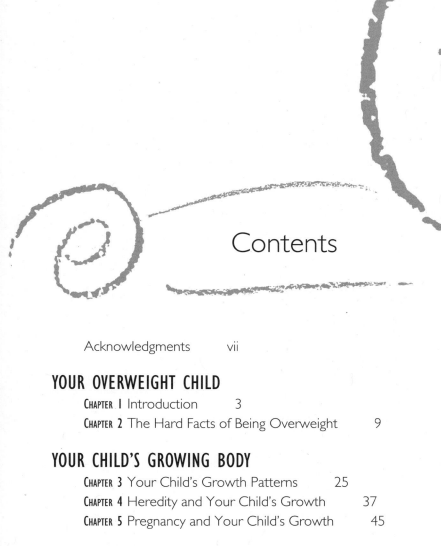

Contents

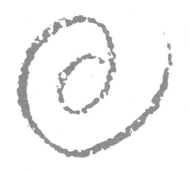

Acknowledgments

*T*hank you—to all my patients and my family and friends for sharing your stories, concerns, and sage advice with me. The patient stories are based on real problems that I have seen in my work, with names and details changed to protect the individuals. I often see the same challenges occurring again and again—so the stories are usually combinations of several patients to further keep my patients' confidentiality.

My family and friends were very tolerant of my calling them up and quizzing them on "what do you do when. . . ." For this, and for their great responses and contributions, I am grateful.

This book is the effort of a group of caring and resourceful people. Jennifer Buechner, RD, CSP, pediatric nutrition specialist at Children's Healthcare of Atlanta, coauthored Chapter 11 with me on the roles and responsibilities of parents and children and was one of my top supporters in getting this written. Thank you to Cathy McCarroll, MPH, RD, LD, instructor in the Division of Nutrition of Georgia State University (formerly with Emory Children's Center), and Xiomara Hinson, nutrition research assistant at Emory Children's Center, who shared their experiences and helped me find answers. Cathy also coordinated the testing of the recipes. Many thanks to Georgia State University nutrition graduate students, Malia Chang, Jennifer DeLuca, Eric Green, Julia Kitromelides, Laurie Ledford, Christine Malek, Rachel Reeves, Ellen Stokes, Mark Stutzman, and Gail Thomas, who prepared and taste-tested the recipes contributed by chefs and parents. Thank you to the students who contributed to the nutrition section of this book: Malia Chang, Jennifer DeLuca, Amber Johnson, and Rachel Reeves. I am grateful to Julie Shaffer, the Slow Food Network coordinator for Atlanta, who urged her many culinary friends to share their recipes and food ideas with me.

A very special thank you to my mother, Cornelia Vanderkooy-Vos, PhD, who answered the many questions "For the Psychologist" from parents that are found throughout the book. She also shared her wisdom on parenting by writing Chapter 15. As one of her five children, I can attest to the soundness of her advice.

Special thanks to the reviewers of the galleys, who provided many insightful suggestions and helpful comments: Ben Gold, MD; Colin Howden, MD, AGAF; Angela Lemond, RD, LD; Melissa Palmer, MD; and Ellyn Satter, MS, RD, LCSW, BCD.

A portion of the proceeds of this book go to the Weight and Wellness Research Fund at Children's Healthcare of Atlanta, where we continue to research ways to prevent, treat, and cure childhood obesity and its related diseases.

MIRIAM B. VOS, MD, MSPH

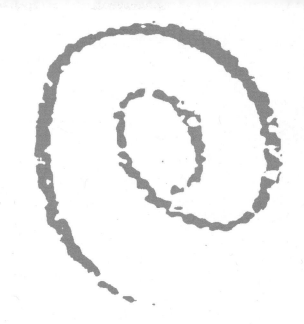

Your Overweight Child

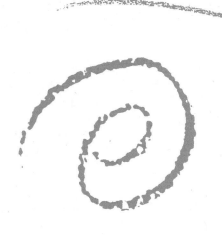

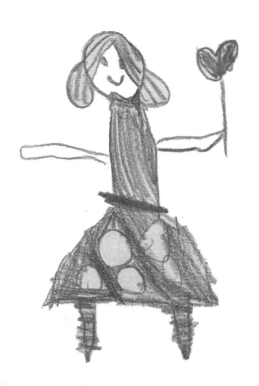

Introduction

One of my physician friends said to me recently, "I don't know what to do. My pediatrician said that my 6-year-old daughter is overweight. And I agree that she is a little chubby. But then Dr. K told me *not* to put her on a diet . . . but that we needed to *make changes*. What does that mean? What do we change?"

We are in the midst of an obesity epidemic. Maybe you picked up this book because your child is overweight. Or maybe you are worried that your child is at risk for obesity. People of all ages are heavier now than just 20 or 30 years ago, but the increase in the number of overweight children is the scariest. Our children are developing serious diseases that typically only occur in adults. For the first time in our nation's history, children cannot expect to have a longer lifespan than their parents.[1] If your family is like the ones I see in clinic, your son or daughter may be on track to develop type 2 diabetes, high blood pressure, or liver disease in their teen years!

If you worry about your child's weight, you are not alone. Scientists, medical professionals, educators, policy makers, and parents like you are increasingly worried that so many of our country's youth are overweight. In my work as a pediatric gastroenterologist, I care for children and teens with digestion, liver, and nutrition problems. I meet a lot of overweight children and their families. My heart goes out to these families, and in my clinic and research work, I have dedicated myself to improving our approach to childhood weight and its complications.

Children Deserve a Different Approach

Children come in all shapes and sizes, but truly healthy children are bright-eyed, able-bodied, energetic, and glowing. They are meant to grow and gain weight at a stable pace. So, how do you get there—what do you do? I am willing to bet that most of what you have heard are things like "exercise 3 times a week for 30 minutes," "control those portion sizes," "eat more celery," and "get on the treadmill." This kind of information is everywhere but these approaches were developed for adults. I find that many physicians know more about adult weight and nutrition than how to help children. One of my patients once brought along a prescription from his pediatrician that read, "Eat carrots and celery 2 times a day." Do these "adult approaches" work for kids? I don't think so!

Children are not just little adults. Their bodies are developing and growing taller and creating the foundation for a long healthy life. The art of improving the health of your children begins with understanding that your child lives in a family. What happens at home in your family is shaped by your history, where you live, and the habits you've developed or slipped into. How you feed your child and your child's relationship with food are shaped by your own experiences with food. Our society has changed over time, and there are pressures on all sides that affect your child. How physically active your child can be at school is largely determined by teachers, administrators, and state policies. In our culture, food is readily available everywhere we go. The advertisers teach our children that we need to eat more of the special foods that they promise will make us happy and entertain us.

For you as a parent, feeding is not just about getting calories and nutrients into the body, it is how we nurture our children and show our love. These connections are behind why it is extra difficult when food and eating become sources of distress and unhealthiness. Can you remember how it was with your new baby? Feeding your infant was top priority—and not always very easy. When I see a baby in my clinic who isn't gaining weight very well, I have to sort out what is happening without increasing the distress of the parents. It's an especially hard task because of the very emotional connection. If I am not careful, I quickly have tearful parents and a crying baby in my office!

Getting Off Track

One of my patients, a 9-year-old named Chris, is a good example of what can happen to any of us. His mom explained that, although Chris was a big baby, during his toddler years he got taller and slimmer and stayed that way. When Chris was 5 years old, his family moved from their apartment to a house. Chris started kindergarten, got his own room, and started playing video games—all at about the same time. His new school was

very good academically, with special music and language programs, but recess time was limited, and physical education (PE)
programs had been reduced. The apartment had been smaller,
so Chris had played outside with other children in the apartment complex. But in the new neighborhood, they didn't know
as many people. Chris's mom went back to work, and she
stopped having as much energy and time to cook. They began
eating out more often or bringing dinner home from one of the
convenient restaurants they passed on the way home. Chris
watched more TV (now he had one in his bedroom), and he
started asking for specific foods and sugary drinks that he spot-
ted in the enticing advertisements.

All of this combined to put Chris on the path of rapid
weight gain. Both his mom and dad were overweight—but for
them it had developed in their 20s and 30s. I think they were
both a little surprised to have a 9-year-old son who was now
inching toward 175 pounds. And, as Chris's mom explained,
"Chris can't keep up with his playmates. He gets short of
breath at football practice, and then he feels bad. We want to
make a change so he can be the best that he can be."

The good news is that Chris's family chose to gradually
make some small but important changes—changes that were
manageable and sustainable. And over time, Chris's health has
improved significantly. At the last visit, Chris told me that he
is stronger and keeps up better with his friends. And, as his
mom pointed out, "You don't see it on the scale, but he is
slimming down through the middle."

Changes that Worked

The first thing that Chris's mother chose to work on was to
start walking three times a week for 15 minutes herself. I know
this seems a little strange, because wasn't it Chris who had the
"problem"? It turns out that parents are the best role models
for children. By resetting the importance of outdoor time in her
own life, she was not just telling Chris to do something different, she was showing him—leading by example. Chris chose to

start riding his bike after school instead of playing video games (in part because his parents were now limiting his time on the games), and it turned out that he liked to bike alongside and around his mother as she walked. After they developed this new habit, they started working on other areas one by one. Chris's dad gave up sodas and started drinking water. This meant that they stopped buying soda and drink boxes on a regular basis. They started cooking more at home. They walked over to a nearby park together on the weekends. These changes didn't happen overnight, but then, Chris didn't gain his weight overnight.

A Better Path

In this book, you will find practical advice, stories, and examples of other families and children and the knowledge you need to navigate the paths of raising your healthy child. There are healthy practices that can help you and your family live more energetic, active lives. There are ways to provide healthy meals despite your busy life. I encourage you to feed your family in a way that makes food a comfortable and nurturing part of your child's life. An important part of being healthy for a child is being comfortable and satisfied with food and eating, both in the family environment and in society. You don't want your son or daughter to feel bad when they think about food. You want them to be a healthy weight for their body *and* full of energy *and* proud of who they are.

Is the Goal to Have Skinny Kids?

No. Kids and families come in all shapes and sizes. Your child's healthy weight may or may not mean a thin body. A child is at a healthy weight when he or she is physically active, has positive relationships with food, and is growing normally. The goal is to have family practices that promote a healthy weight for all members of the family over the long term.

This is not a diet book full of quick fix promises. This is not a special program that you do for a few weeks. It's a new approach that can change you, your children, and perhaps the world around you. Think about your family and your own habits. Are your current habits promoting a healthy life for you? For your child? I hope that you will find in the chapters and examples ahead ideas and inspiration to start making some small changes that will lead you all down a new path to healthier lives.

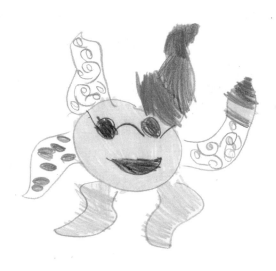

2

The Hard Facts
of Being Overweight

Children come to see me because they have developed a disease or condition that is caused by being overweight or obese. Here are some facts about those unhealthy conditions. Childhood obesity can do a lot of damage. My hope is that this information gives you more good reasons to make changes to improve your child's health.

> ## Health Problems Caused by Obesity in Children
>
> **Physical problems**
> - Impaired balance and athletic abilities
> - Joint pain and injuries (orthopedic problems)
> - Insulin resistance and prediabetes
> - Type 2 diabetes
> - High blood pressure (hypertension)
> - High cholesterol and high triglycerides
> - Nonalcoholic fatty liver disease
> - Gallstones
> - Sleep apnea (snoring and difficulty breathing while asleep)
>
> **Emotional problems**
> - Low self-esteem
> - Negative body image
> - Depression
>
> **Social problems**
> - Being singled out as different
> - Feeling rejected by other children
> - Being discriminated against
> - Being teased and bullied
> - Being left out of most social groups
>
> _____
>
> *Source:* Reference 2.

When we eat, our body directs the food energy to different places. Some gets used right away. Some gets stored for later use in the "short-term storage tanks." Some gets sent for long-term storage as fat deposits located just under the skin. In overnutrition, too much energy gets stored as fats in "storage tanks" around the thighs, waist, and elsewhere. Although a small amount of stored fat is good, large fat deposits stress the body.

A variety of problems tend to occur when the body has too much fat. But most often, my young patients have joint/bone damage, prediabetes or type 2 diabetes, high blood pressure, fatty liver disease, and social problems, like being bullied at school.

You may have heard of the metabolic syndrome (also called syndrome X or the dysmetabolic syndrome). Metabolic syndrome is not a disease itself but a collection of changes that can occur in the body as we become overweight. Doctors use this collection of changes to gauge how much a person is affected by weight gain, especially to estimate the future risk of heart disease.

> **Characteristics of the Metabolic Syndrome**
>
> ☺ Increased waist circumference
> ☺ Hypertension
> ☺ High cholesterol
> ☺ High triglycerides
> ☺ Type 2 diabetes

How weight gain affects health varies widely. Some of my patients weigh 300 pounds or more and have normal cholesterol levels and normal blood pressure. But Carla, for example, has a different genetic profile. At age 12, she is heavier than average but doesn't meet the technical definition of overweight. (Chapter 3 presents these definitions.) Despite her mild weight gain, she has more fat at her waist (rather than a waist smaller than her hips), high cholesterol, high blood pressure, and a fatty liver. Carla has full-blown metabolic syndrome. Genetically, she is less tolerant of weight gain.

Prediabetes and Type 2 Diabetes

Type 2 diabetes is basically a disease of the overweight—especially in children. Type 2 usually develops in older adults, but with the obesity epidemic, it increasingly occurs in children. Taking in too much energy from food day in and day out puts high demands on the insulin system.

Insulin is a hormone made in the pancreas and released in response to eating. Food is turned into glucose that circulates in the bloodstream. Insulin's job is to move glucose from the bloodstream to cells that can either use it as fuel or store it for later. Each cell that uses glucose, such as liver, muscle, and fat cells, has receptors (like docking stations) for insulin. When insulin joins with an insulin receptor, it allows the glucose to leave the blood and enter these cells.

Normal Action of Insulin

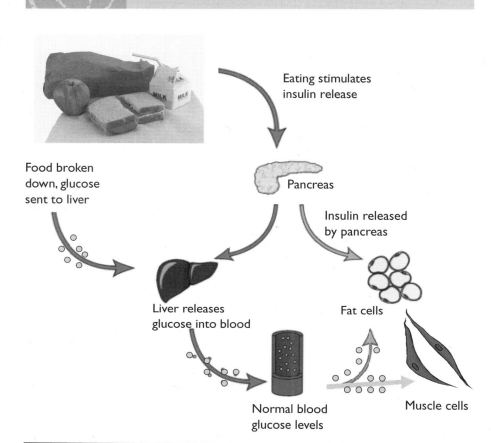

Eating stimulates insulin release

Food broken down, glucose sent to liver

Pancreas

Insulin released by pancreas

Liver releases glucose into blood

Fat cells

Normal blood glucose levels

Muscle cells

Source: Adapted from www.endocrineweb.com/insulin.html. Accessed December 22, 2008.

In the condition called *prediabetes,* your child's insulin receptors become less sensitive to insulin. This condition is called *insulin resistance* because insulin receptors resist the insulin. The body deals with this by making extra insulin to flood the receptors. The body needs more and more insulin to control glucose levels. Over time, the pancreas cannot keep up with the demand and "burns out." Glucose levels rise and stay above normal, which is defined as type 2 diabetes.

Combining daily physical activity with eating changes is the best treatment to stop prediabetes from becoming type 2 diabetes. This is also the way to manage type 2 diabetes if you already have it. In addition, you may need either medications that help the cells become sensitive to insulin again or to inject insulin if your body can't make enough.

A common sign of insulin resistance is called *acanthosis nigricans*. This darkening of the skin can look like dirt that doesn't wash off, most often near the base of the neck. This condition improves or even disappears if insulin and glucose levels return to normal.

Insulin resistance and type 2 diabetes are different from type 1 diabetes, where the child's body stops making any insulin at all. But both types of diabetes cause high blood glucose and have the same symptoms. Be sure to have your child's blood glucose level checked by your pediatrician if your child is:

- excessively thirsty
- urinating frequently (especially getting up frequently at night)
- unusually tired

High Blood Pressure

Most children have normal blood pressure. But overweight children can have high blood pressure (also called *hypertension*). Over time, increased pressure damages the circulatory system and can lead to heart attacks and strokes. Developing hypertension earlier in life than usual can run in families, and if it does in yours, your child is at increased risk. Your child's blood pressure should be checked at each well child check-up, so ask your pediatrician to tell you your child's blood pressure. Sometimes, the result can be wrong if your child is nervous or the blood pressure cuff is too big or too small. A diagnosis of hypertension should not be based on a single high reading. But if it is high once, you should return to the office to have it rechecked.

All of the healthy changes in this book will help if your child has hypertension, but several are recommended specifically for hypertension:

- lose weight or stop weight gain (keep weight level)

⊚ eat more vegetables and fruits

⊚ eat low-salt foods and stop adding salt to food '

High Cholesterol and High Triglycerides (Hyperlipidemia)

By the age of 7, children's blood fat levels begin to have the same patterns seen in adults. Children who are overweight often have higher than normal levels of the two main blood fats that are associated with increased risk of heart disease: cholesterol and triglycerides. Your child's pediatrician will track this with blood tests. High cholesterol and high triglycerides (together called *hyperlipidemia*) tend to run in families because of inherited genes that increase (or fail to remove) cholesterol and triglycerides in the blood.

Cholesterol is a fat that is mostly made by the liver. A small amount of cholesterol is absorbed from our food (from animal products) as well. Triglycerides are a form of stored energy, and the levels rise immediately after a meal. Certain foods signal the body to make more triglycerides. For example, eating a meal that is high in fat or high in fructose (a common sugar in food) causes high blood triglyceride levels that last several hours or longer after meals. For this reason, in addition to physical activity, treatment of this condition includes avoiding foods with high fat or high sugar levels.

Cholesterol and triglyceride levels often normalize with weight loss and physical activity. If not, there are a variety of effective medications that help. If the levels do not improve with increased activity and improved nutrition, medications should be used starting in the teenage years.

Nonalcoholic Fatty Liver Disease (NAFLD)

Fatty liver develops in some children who are overweight. Fat is not normally stored in the liver, except in animals who are getting ready to migrate or hibernate. In humans, fat is stored in the liver if there is a problem with fat regulation: too much is coming in to the liver or not enough can be shipped out.

Fatty liver or NAFLD (non-alcoholic fatty liver disease) can be very mild, with just some extra fat, or it can be severe, where inflammation and scar tissue develop in the liver along with the fat. NAFLD has no obvious symptoms. Your pediatrician may feel your child's abdomen to know whether the liver is too big or use a blood test to check liver enzymes. The severe form of fatty liver is called *nonalcoholic steatohepatitis* (NASH). Over years, NASH can scar the liver so badly that it stops functioning well, a condition called *cirrhosis*.

NAFLD seems to run in families and occurs more often in children who have parents and grandparents with type 2 diabetes. In the United States, overweight white and Latino children have a higher risk of getting fatty liver than overweight African American children. This is probably because of genetic inheritance patterns but could be related to shared lifestyles and habits. The best way for your child to avoid developing fatty liver disease is to play outside, get lots of exercise, and avoid sugar-sweetened beverages. NAFLD can improve when your child becomes healthier.

Gallstones

Obese children are more likely to develop gallstones, which are hardened bits of cholesterol and bile salts inside the gallbladder that normally aren't present. The gallbladder is a small storage organ that is attached to the main drainage "pipe" of the liver. It stores bile from the liver. Although the connection between obesity and gallstones is not clear, when bile is high in cholesterol, gallstones are more likely to form.

Although gallstones themselves are not a problem, people who have them can pass one or more out of the gallbladder when it releases bile. Bile helps us digest food, especially the fats in food. After an especially fatty meal, such as a large hamburger or steak, extra bile is released from the gallbladder to help digest the extra fat. When released, bile from the gallbladder can take a stone with it. The stone can create irritation as it passes through the duct leading into the small intestine, or the stone can block the duct. Typically, this causes severe right-sided pain a few hours after eating. If your child has had this kind of pain after a meal, speak to your pediatrician. Gallstones are found by abdominal ultrasound and can be treated in various ways, including gallbladder removal.

Sleep Apnea

Children who are overweight have increased risk of breathing problems when sleeping.[3] They are more likely to snore, and they are five times more likely to develop obstructive sleep apnea. Obstructive sleep apnea is when both breathing and sleep are interrupted multiple times by a partial or complete blockage of the airway. The airway can be narrowed by excess neck flesh or by large tonsils in the throat.

Sleep apnea at night makes a child very tired during the day. When a healthy child sleeps, you'll hear deep and regular breathing. With sleep apnea, there will be a pause between breaths. The pause can seem too long, and often breathing will begin again suddenly, usually along with the child moving around in bed. The child is actually waking up a little to change position to start breathing again.

To diagnose sleep apnea, your child will need to spend a night sleeping in a lab monitored by sensors for breathing. If your child has sleep apnea, there are ways to ensure regular breathing with the aid of a machine, weight loss, or possibly surgery.

Not all children who are overweight need a sleep study.[4] But important warning signs that you should discuss with your doctor are

- you notice that your child has periods of interrupted breathing (apnea) while sleeping
- your child has restless sleep and seems tired on waking most mornings

◎ you know your child has large tonsils or your doctor
finds large tonsils

Joint and Bone Damage

Consider a boy who is 5 feet, 4 inches tall and weighs 200
pounds. His body was "meant" to be closer to 125 pounds. His
bones have to carry the extra weight all the time, just as though
he always has on a backpack with 75 pounds of books in it.

Extra weight causes stress and inflammation in the hips
and knees. The most common hip problem in adolescents usually occurs during adolescent growth spurts, but can also occur
in obese younger children. The ball of bone that rests in the hip
socket gradually slides out of place on the top of the femoral
bone (called *slipped capital femoral epiphysis or SCFE*).[5] The
displacement can happen because of a build up of normal
forces over time or it can happen suddenly as an injury. If the
injury is gradual—the pain can have been there for a while,
even months. If the ball slips off, it needs emergency surgical
repair so it's important to get diagnosed. This problem is painful,
but the pain isn't always in the hip; it can be in the groin, knee,
or thigh, so it can be difficult to diagnose. Pain in any of these
locations, especially if it causes your child to limp, should
always be investigated by a doctor.

Blount's disease is another bone problem in which the
lower legs begin to bow. Although it's normal for a toddler to
have a bow-legged appearance, this should improve between
the ages of 2 and 4 years. But in Blount's disease, which is
associated with obesity, the bowing of the legs gets worse over
time. Excess body weight makes the condition worse.

Excess weight can cause general increased stress on all the
joints. Obviously, children with joint pain are not likely to enjoy
running in a soccer game or participating in sports. One challenge will be to find activities that do not increase the joint pain
but provide a way for the child to use up extra calories so that
they can reduce the strain on their joints. Consider swimming
or bike riding.

Emotional Problems

Being overweight can affect your child's long-term mood and outlook. Several studies have shown that overweight children are more likely to have anxiety, depression, and eating disorders than their normal-weight peers.[6–8] Each child deals with this in his or her own way. Some have low self-esteem in general, while others show strong self-esteem in some areas but low body self-esteem. Many overweight children are not bothered at all.

Symptoms of depression in teenagers can be subtle. They may seem tired and more irritable. They may increase or decrease their sleep or their eating from what is normal. They may isolate themselves or cry more than usual. Most children with depression will deny that they feel depressed, so asking them isn't really a good way to diagnose it. If you are concerned that your child may be depressed or have other emotional problems, your pediatrician can refer you to a counselor or psychologist who can evaluate your child.

School Performance Problems

Can being overweight affect your child's ability to learn? In fact, your overweight child may not be performing up to his or her full potential. One study looked at the academic and cognitive functioning of more than 2,500 children with an average age of 12 years and compared this to their body mass index (BMI).[9] BMI is a measure of weight that takes into account height. There is more about BMI in Chapter 3.

In this study, researchers found that there were no differences in the reading or math test scores earned by children when grouped by BMI. However, overweight children did not do as well on a "block-design" test, which measures cognitive functioning. In this test, the child is asked to make a copy of a two-dimensional geometric pattern using a set of three-dimensional cubes. This measures the child's ability to reason and to accurately create a model of something seen as a picture (visual-spacial construction ability). As BMI went up, the scores on the block-design test went down. This was true whether the child came from a high- or low-income family or had highly educated parents or not.

The authors of this study wondered if these differences could be related to sleep problems, like obstructive sleep apnea, or to changes in insulin levels or other hormones. They point out that, "Today's schools face intense pressure to focus on standardized tests and consequently have placed less emphasis on the broader view of a healthy mind in a healthy body." As a parent, you can make your voice heard at your child's school about the importance of increasing physical activity, which helps all the children perform better. Kids 4 to 18 years old who are more physically active have better perceptual skills, achievement, verbal tests, mathematical tests, academic readiness, and intelligence.[10] And, increased physical activity in schools helps prevent and protect your child from gaining too much weight.

Social Problems

For the overweight child and teen, social problems are more a part of daily life than illness. Children can be very cruel. Teasing and bullying unfortunately occurs often among adolescents, but overweight teens and children are targeted because they are seen as different and undesirable. Being teased about weight is painful and can increase your child's feelings of failure and inadequacy. This kind of treatment lowers their self-esteem. Teasing and negative comments by other children may even lead to depression.[11] Depression and poor self-esteem can make it hard for children to want to get involved with others, or even go outside to play or exercise. Social isolation, poor self-esteem, and depression contribute to low activity levels and poor eating habits. And this makes the obesity worse—a vicious cycle. Overweight children are less likely to go to college and to succeed. This kind of future is scary and not what you desire for your child.

What can you do? First, you can help your child identify these harmful events as "harmful." Some bullying is obvious, like name calling on the playground that happens in elementary school. In high school, bullying can be less obvious but just as painful. It hurts to be gossiped about or excluded from groups and invitations. It hurts not to have good friends.[12]

- Ask your child about school and interactions with others. Use broad, open-ended questions, such as, "Is there anything that made you feel upset today?"
- Help your child see the bullying for what it is: bad behavior on someone else's part. It's important that your child realizes that it is not his or her fault. No one deserves to be ridiculed.
- Encourage your child to seek positive relationships at school. Friends are the best protection against being bullied and becoming a bully. Being in a group is a natural way children protect themselves from being singled out.
- Help your child connect with other children with whom he or she can play or share a hobby and have fun. This may be outside of school—maybe at the local community center or in your neighborhood.
- Talk with your child about how to handle teasing when it happens and encourage him or her to ignore it and walk away. Getting upset or reacting to the teasing only encourages the other child to continue. Sometimes a single firm statement will deflect the bully, such as, "You're boring me" or "Go somewhere else."
- Take your concerns about bad treatment of your child to the school principal, nurse, or counselor. Work with them over the school year.
- Consider counseling sessions with or for your child to help him or her figure out ways to cope.
- Spending time with your child will show how important and special he or she is and will help him or her develop the inner strength and resilience to deal with life's ups and downs (like bullying).

Don't ever give up. Compared to adults, children have the best chance to improve their weight, especially if they are still growing taller. As a family, you have the opportunity to feel better and enjoy being healthier if you take small, manageable steps toward healthier living.

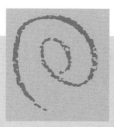

Question for the Psychologist

Q **My daughter is 15 years old, weighs 260 pounds, and has very few friends. She is teased at school. It's getting so bad that I think she might drop out. How do I help her? Should I go to the principal or the teachers?**

A I feel for you both. Being teased and feeling rejected by peers is a harsh and painful experience. The two of you probably cannot fix this by yourselves. Talk to the school guidance counselor about the teasing. Schedule an appointment with a child psychologist who can help your daughter figure out how to deal with the teasing, suggest ways to improve her social skills, and provide support in developing healthier lifestyle habits. You might help your daughter find hobbies or develop talents, such as singing or acting, that will provide her a natural way to interact with others.

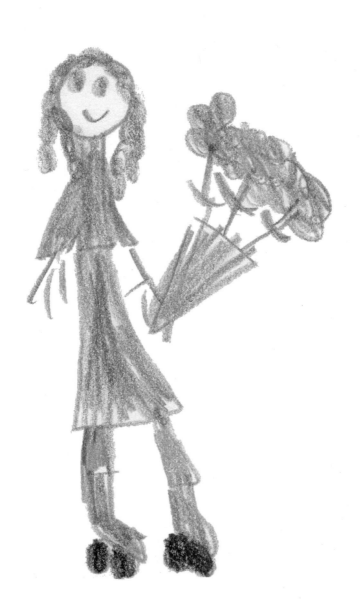

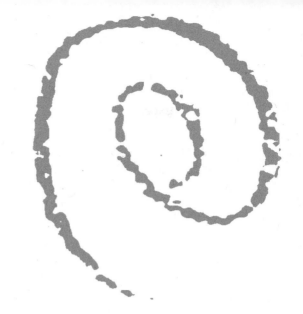

Your Child's Growing Body

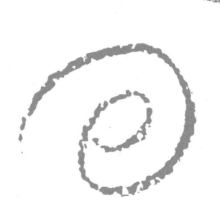

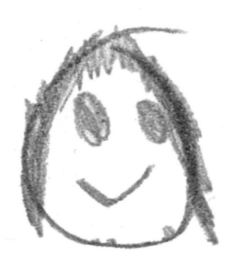

3

Your Child's
Growth Patterns

When Sam was born, he was very long and thin. He was born a few weeks early, and the delivery was difficult—resulting in a large bruise on his head. After some recovery days in the hospital nursery, he went home with his mother. Breastfeeding was difficult at first because he didn't want to latch on. His first visit with the pediatrician was worrisome because he had lost weight. But within a week, he began to get better at feeding and breastfed around the clock. At six months, Sam was still exclusively breastfed and was a very fat baby. He had three chins! Even strangers would comment on what a big baby he was.

Although the change was a little shocking, his mother knew that breastfed babies can be trusted to control their own caloric intake. All through his first year, he was "off the chart" for both height and weight. By age 2, he was running all over the house, yard, and nearby parks. His body started to slim down. Now age 7, he has become a great little soccer player, bike rider, and swimmer. He is muscular and not overweight at all.

We know that most children fit into some typical patterns of growth. Sam's pattern is one pattern that is seen for breastfed babies. Breastfed babies tend to have a slower start gaining weight but some become much fatter between 6 and 12 months old. On average, breastfed babies are thinner than formula-fed babies, and from toddler years on, breastfed children have less chance of being overweight. These patterns of growing are averages that researchers and physicians have put together by studying large groups of children.

Do you feel pressure to raise a child who is the "right" size and shape? How much control do you have over what size and shape your child ends up being?

Height and weight gain are determined by two main influences: genetics and the environment. Genetics is the part that we don't control. It's the hand that we are dealt. But, we do get to choose what we do with what we are given. The environment reflects those choices, from how physically active we are to what we eat—and when we eat it. In this chapter, I will explain how doctors measure growth in children, what is "normal," and how to work with what you have inherited.

How Growth Happens

In the first year of life, the average baby triples its weight. By two years of age, most children have reached half of their adult height. It takes 15 or so years to gain the other half.

I like to call Sam my "first baby" because I learned a lot watching him and his mother Catherine. One of the things she pointed out was that as an infant, sometimes Sam would eat all day long. He couldn't get enough. And a few days later, she noticed that he was longer! Other times, especially when he was around 2 years old, he wouldn't eat much at all, and his clothes would fit for a long time.

What Catherine was seeing is real. Michelle Lampl's research shows that children grow in bursts, even over hours, followed by long periods of no growth. This challenges traditional thinking in the medical community that children have constant growth.[13] This is why the smooth curving lines on standard growth charts may not represent how growth occurs in a unique individual like your child.

Because infants grow so rapidly, their growth spurts are even more striking. Dr. Lampl followed nine breastfed infants over the first year of life, measuring them every week. When she plotted the growth of one baby girl on the chart, at times it looked like she was lagging behind by 25% compared to what she should have gained. But a week later, she had caught up. The figure below shows how a real baby boy and girl grow, with much more variation than the smooth dotted lines

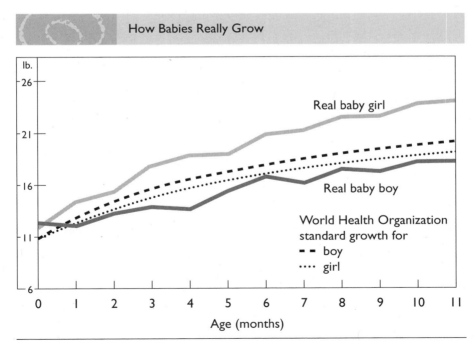

Source: Adapted from Reference 13.

that the World Health Organization uses to show standard growth.

In medicine, our concept of what and how much a baby needs to eat is based on old ideas that children grow a little bit each and every day. But Sam's mom was right. Sam eats more sometimes and grows more sometimes. Growth spurts lead to "bursts of eating" as well.

Children are born knowing how much food they need for energy each day. It's important to trust this and not press them to finish the bottle or eat another jar of baby food just because that is how much they "usually" eat. Pediatricians are learning to give infants a chance to follow their own unique growth pattern and not be so concerned about how they compare with the growth charts. Unfortunately, being "underweight" or "overweight" at a check-up can put pressure on you to change your child's natural desire to eat. If you pressure your children to eat more or to eat less, you can harm their inborn eating patterns. I'll talk more about this in Chapter 11.

Older children grow in different ways, too. Some gain weight and look a little stout, and then they seem to thin out overnight by growing taller. Others follow a smooth transition in height and weight and appear to keep the same proportions for years. Many boys spend years looking up to their female schoolmates only to gain several inches of height in time for high school graduation. These individual differences are difficult to capture on "standardized" growth charts.

Tracking Growth Patterns

The doctor tracks your child's growth by checking height and weight regularly and recording these on standardized charts. Pay attention to the *pattern* your child has already shown. This is the most important trend because it is unique to your child.

Look at Sam's growth chart. Because he was a few weeks premature, he gained weight rapidly in the first few months to "catch up" with his height. Most babies gain fat during the last few weeks of gestation, and Sam missed out on this by being

Sam's First Year

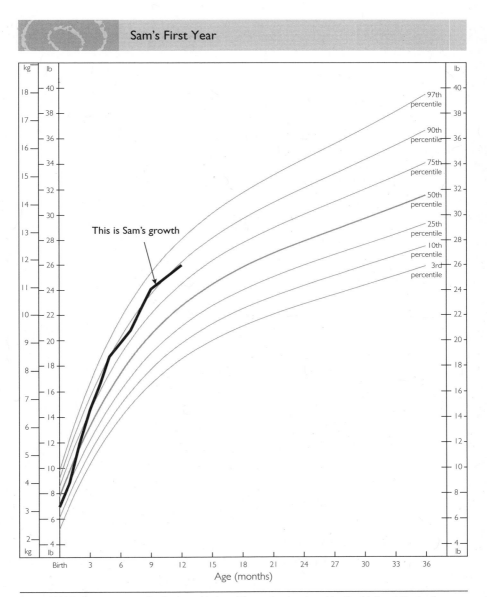

Source: Weight-for-age percentiles for boys, birth to 36 months, developed by the National Center for Health Statistics in collaboration with the National Center for Chronic Disease Prevention and Health Promotion (2000).

born early. You can see that he doesn't follow the "average lines." In fact, he crosses them and shoots up the 95th percentile for weight—which matches his height. At times he is even above the top of the chart. All of this is normal growth for Sam.

Weight Definitions for Children	
Weight Category	**Percentile Range**
Underweight	Less than the 5th percentile
Healthy weight	5th percentile to less than the 85th percentile
Overweight	85th percentile to less than the 95th percentile
Obese	95th percentile and over

Source: www.cdc.gov/nccdphp/dnpa/healthyweight/assessing/bmi/childrens_BMI/about_childrens_BMI.htm. Accessed October 8, 2008.

I want you to be familiar with growth charts when your child's pediatrician uses them, but I also want to put in a word of caution. The charts were made by collecting the heights and weights of 10,000 American children at one point in time. Does this make a difference? Yes, it does. The real growth and weight gain of an individual child are not nearly as smooth as the lines on the chart.

Height

Your child's doctor will measure height at each well child check-up. By putting your child's height on the growth chart by age, the pediatrician can compare your child's growth to the average for children in the United States. There are different charts for boys and for girls by age: children birth to 36 months and children age 2 to 20 years.

Take a look at the height chart for boys age 2 to 20 years. The middle line is the 50th percentile, which is the average child's height by age. The lines below this middle line show the pattern for a shorter-than-average child, one who would fall in the 10th or 25th percentiles. The lines above the middle line show the pattern for a taller-than-average child.

Height Chart for a Tall Boy

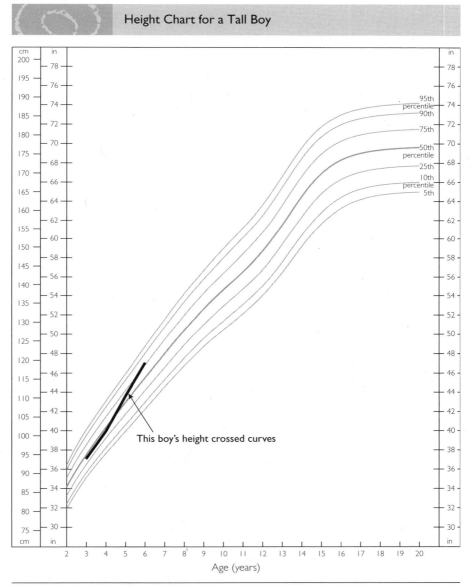

This boy's height crossed curves

Source: Stature-for-age percentiles for boys, 2 to 20 years, developed by the National Center for Health Statistics in collaboration with the National Center for Chronic Disease Prevention and Health Promotion (2000).

If a child is growing faster than average, his measurements will be above the line. It is typical for children of tall parents to be in the 95th percentile. Some genetic conditions cause growth that is below average. There is a different growth chart for children born with Down's syndrome because they grow more slowly.

Weight

Doctors also track children's weight on standardized charts. But unlike height, weight can go up or down due to illness and other events. Take a look at the weight gain pattern of a breastfed infant. This child's growth did not exactly follow the smooth line of the average child's weight gain—and this is not surprising because each child is unique! At the next check-up, ask your doctor to show you the pattern your child has been following for height and weight changes.

You need to know your child's height and weight compared to the patterns that he or she has already shown. If your child's weight pretty much followed the same pattern for the first five years of life but in the past six months has shot way above average, you and your doctor need to look for the reasons why that is happening.

Keep in mind two important points about these charts:

⚲ There is no one "right" height and weight for a child of a particular age.
⚲ Although it's tempting to use the charts to predict your child's future height and weight, this cannot be done with absolute certainty.

Body Mass Index

After age 2, your child's doctor will begin to record another measurement called *body mass index* (BMI). BMI is a measure that uses both height and weight in a formula to show how they relate to each other.

$$\left[weight(lb) / height(in)^2 \right] \times 703$$

Normal Growth for a Breastfed Infant

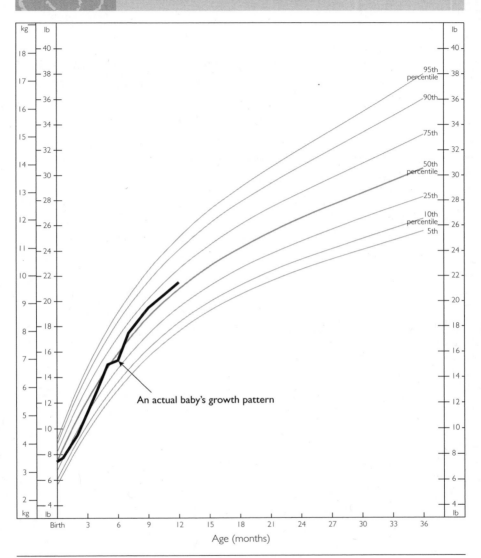

Source: Weight-for-age percentiles for girls, birth to 36 months, developed by the National Center for Health Statistics in collaboration with the National Center for Chronic Disease Prevention and Health Promotion (2000).

BMI is the common method for estimating whether a child's (or an adult's) weight matches his or her height. The doctor plots your child's BMI on a growth chart used by the Centers for Disease Control (CDC). Like the charts for height and weight, this one was designed using the averages of BMI measurements in thousands of children of different ages.

There are different charts for girls and boys, by age. A BMI in the 60th percentile means that the child's BMI is higher than 60% of other children of the same age and sex. Because adults have stopped growing, there are fixed cutoffs for BMI rather than percentiles.

You can use the CDC's BMI calculators at **www.cdc.gov/nccdphp/dnpa/bmi/index.htm** to determine BMIs for your entire family by age.

BMI changes as children grow. It usually decreases between ages 2 and 6 and then increases, leveling off at adulthood. If a child gains weight faster than he or she grows in height, the BMI will increase, whether the child is gaining muscle or fat.

A very muscular child will often have a BMI higher than most other children but this is not unhealthy. This is because muscle weighs more than fat. Boys and girls have different amounts of body fat at different ages, and the charts take this into account.

Interpreting the Charts for Your Child

The best use of the height, weight, and BMI charts is to see the pattern of your child's growth over time. Has it been stable (following a curve), or is it rising or falling above and below the standard lines? Have your child's weight and height both increased or is one way ahead of the other? How does your child's growth compare with other boys or girls the same age? Talk with your pediatrician about your child's individual growing trends.

A Child with BMI Rising Across Percentiles

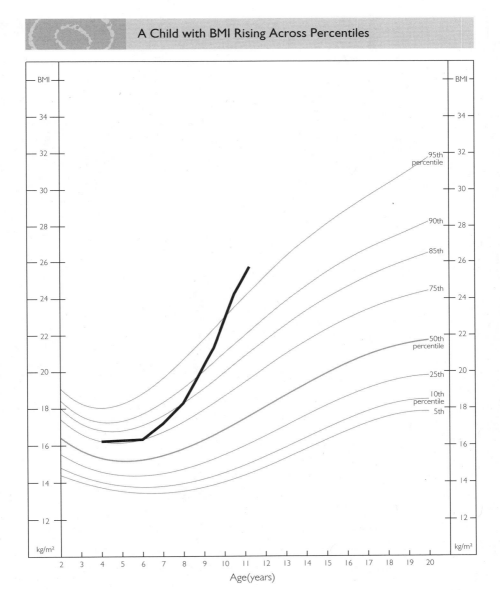

Source: Body mass index-for-age percentiles for girls, 2 to 20 years, developed by the National Center for Health Statistics in collaboration with the National Center for Chronic Disease Prevention and Health Promotion (2000).

Over time, the BMI of a child who is gaining more weight than height will begin to "rise across percentiles." Crossing lines does not necessarily mean that your child is overweight, but it can be *a warning sign* about your child's health.

The CDC's Nutrition Division considers a child with a BMI above the 85th percentile to be overweight and those above the 95th percentile to be obese. In the United States, one in six children is considered obese by this definition. Keep in mind that a child's change in growth pattern is more important than the percentile. What about your child? What do you know about his or her growth from the height, weight, and BMI charts? Is now the time to make some healthy changes in your family's daily habits?

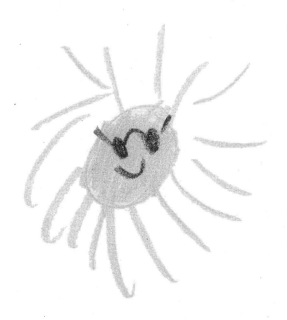

Heredity and
Your Child's Growth

4

At Juan's 11-year-old well check-up, his mother asked the pediatrician about Juan's risk of diabetes. She and his father both have type 2 diabetes. Juan's weight was at the 90th percentile but his BMI did not indicate that he was overweight. Also, the doctor noticed that Juan had dark patches of skin called *acanthosis nigricans* on his neck, a sign of insulin resistance (see page 13). The doctor did a blood test to check for diabetes and liver problems. Juan's high insulin level indicated that he likely already had prediabetes. He also had high liver enzymes, and he was sent to a specialist who diagnosed Juan with fatty liver disease.

Family Risk of Overweight/Obesity in Children

- If one parent is overweight/obese: Child's risk of being overweight increases by 3 times
- If both parents are overweight/obese: Child's risk of being overweight increases by 13 times

Even though Juan wasn't overweight by the growth chart, he already had at least two complications of obesity: pre-diabetes and fatty liver disease. Because of his genes (two parents with diabetes), Juan's healthy weight is lower than the 90th percentile—maybe closer to the 50th percentile, or even less. So, although the charts didn't show him as "obese," Juan was at an unhealthy weight.

Obesity is a strongly genetic condition. A child with one overweight parent is 3 times more likely to be an overweight adult.[14] Genes have a strong influence, but the food and activity habits that families share are just as strong. Obesity is definitely a family matter.

Genetics Determine Metabolic Flexibility

A colleague recently talked with me about one of our mutual patients, an overweight child. My colleague believed that the child must be eating too much. Every time he came to clinic, the mother would explain that it didn't *seem* like he ate more than his brothers—yet he kept getting bigger. My physician friend thought that maybe the mother was fooling herself and not really keeping track. I agree that to gain weight, a child has to eat more calories than he or she burns. But in my experience, overweight children don't have remarkably bigger appetites. In fact, it can sometimes seem like they eat less than another child of the same age and height.

Another colleague told me about his own son's tremendous appetite. A soccer player in high school, he is eating them "out of house and home." They often stop at a fast food restaurant on the way home from practice to get him a snack and then he eats dinner "again" at home. Other times, if his dad is working late, he will call and ask him to pick up a cheeseburger and fries on the way home for another snack. Assuming this is a regular eating pattern, his son is eating a lot of processed, high-fat foods. If he is a typical high school athlete, he probably drinks a lot of high-sugar sports drinks at the games and practices as well. And yet his son is not overweight; in fact, he is thin. Why?

This boy has two kinds of protection against becoming overweight: a very active lifestyle and genes that provide *metabolic flexibility*. Being active not only burns calories during the activity, it also increases the metabolic rate (how quickly calories are used) of your child's body. The more we exercise, the more muscle cells we build and maintain. These muscle cells burn calories all day long—even when we sleep. The body is constantly remodeling itself, so if we quit using the muscles, they quickly are downsized in response. A good example of this is how many muscular football players gain fat after the season ends. Muscle cells must be used to be maintained. If you stop using them but continue eating like you did when you were active, your body puts the energy into fat—an easy storage form. Your *metabolism* is the rate at which your body uses the food you eat as energy to fuel, grow, and repair your body. A high metabolism (usually an active child with good muscle mass) will burn more calories than a slower metabolism.

Metabolic flexibility explains why some of us better tolerate bad habits than others. To understand metabolic flexibility, it may help to think about a rubber garden hose. If you have a freeze-proof hose made of strong, flexible rubber, and water inside the hose freezes and expands, then the hose expands, too. The system is flexible and protects the hose against damage. But if you happen to have a hose made of thinner, hard rubber, the freezing water expands and cracks the hose. When you start watering again in spring . . . the hose leaks, and you get wet.

Some children and adults have very flexible metabolic systems. They can go through periods when they drink sugary sodas, eat out often, and sit on the couch each evening without doing their health any harm for the short-term. Certainly, most people have enough metabolic flexibility to have occasional "treats" without any long-term harm. Thinking about the soccer player, you can see that the more active your child is, the more flexible his or her metabolism will be as well.

Each child has a threshold—a level at which poor lifestyle habits start to cause problems. For example, eating fries and a hamburger at a restaurant once a week will probably not change your child's health. But eating out two, three, and sometimes, four times a week will crack anyone's metabolism. Most of us would gain weight if we consumed daily fast food and sodas (remember the movie *Supersize Me?*) . . . except maybe a teenage soccer player who practices 4 hours a day, like my colleague's son. But he could become deficient in vitamins, antioxidants, and fiber from a largely fast food diet, so I wouldn't recommend it.

Look at your family. Have any of you developed diseases linked to overnutrition, such as obesity, high blood pressure, type 2 diabetes, or fatty liver disease? If so, it's clear that your family has less metabolic flexibility. This is a warning sign: you need to do some things to balance out these genes. If you want your child to be healthier, you will want to provide an active childhood and commit to good family nutrition.

Genetics and Activity Level

In church one Sunday, I watched a young family sitting two pews in front of me. There were two boys about 3 and 6 years old and a little 2-year-old girl. The littlest one was first standing beside her mother, then she was hanging over the back of the pew, then she was climbing over her mom to pester her brother and then after some instruction, she was back in her mother's lap, for a moment. She was in constant motion. Her brothers both sat and colored in a book quietly. They were a little older and that probably helped them sit still, but the little girl clearly had a different temperament.

If you have several children, you may have noticed big differences in their activity levels even when they were very young. Some mothers can describe differences in how much one baby moved during the pregnancy compared to another. Researchers have studied infants with motion monitors and found that the amount of moving the baby does varies a lot.[15] Studies have also shown that the infants who move less are more likely to end up overweight. This is important information that we can respond to.

Each child is born with a unique set of genes and that includes a unique personality that influences how active he or she is. All children benefit from being active. But some children will need extra help in this area. Other children can't stop moving, running, playing, wiggling, and the like. Those kids won't need much help with being active, except perhaps to make sure the TV is off enough of the time. Even the "best genes" usually can't overcome the attraction of the TV. The point is that you don't get to change your child's personality, but you can respond to it.

I have two cats who are sisters from the same litter. When I went to see the kittens, I had every intention to get just one—the big white one with the brown and orange spots on her head. She was the biggest of the litter and so adorable as she rolled and played in the box in the garage. But as I was watching her, the mamma cat laid down, and all the little kittens pounced on her nipples to feed. One, two, three, all the way to nine kittens—but there were only eight spots to nurse from. One little brown kitten was left out, and it had probably happened before because she was small, thin, and weak. So, I took them both home and spent the first few weeks feeding the little one milk with a syringe. They are both beautiful cats now—more than 14 years old. But Bob has always been bigger. At first, I just thought she was a big housecat. But when she developed diabetes at age 5 and a fatty liver, I had to admit that she truly was overweight. She has always been less active than her sister Reepacheep. It's hard to get Bob to chase anything—not a string or a ball or a feather. She mostly sleeps on my bed. Reepacheep has always been naturally more active and is healthy. They both get the same free access to good quality food. When someone points out how big Bob is, I respond, "I know. I feel terrible about taking her out for fast food all those times."

These two cats have the same environment and at least some of the same genes. Of course, I really didn't feed Bob fast food. But, unfortunately, I didn't realize early enough that Bob didn't need "just the same" environment—she needed more. It took a bit of creativity, but I learned some tricks to help Bob stay as healthy as possible. For example, I put the food for both cats up on a counter, so they have to jump up several levels to get to it—automatic exercise. And I moved the food to a room that is farthest away from the family room, where we hang out the most. These changes did make a difference. If only I had noticed the warning signs earlier (she was sedentary from the beginning), I might have prevented some of the complications and she might have turned out to be as healthy as her sister.

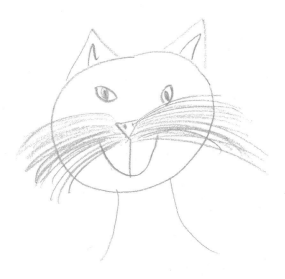

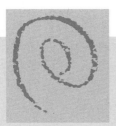

Question for the Psychologist

Q **I am terrified that my kids will end up fat like I was in my teens and twenties. It took me years to learn, but now I can manage my weight. How do I keep from transferring all these feelings of fear to my teenage girl? She is really starting to put on weight.**

A As you have "been there," your daughter will see your actions and words as genuine. Be positive about yourself. You are a courageous person who has overcome great difficulties with weight. You did not give up in spite of many discouraging experiences. You persisted, chose to make changes, and now are successfully living a new lifestyle. You are a strong model for your daughter of continuing to cope with challenges and trying to do what it takes to be healthy.

Sit down and ask your daughter if she is worried about her weight gain. Listen to her concerns. Don't interrupt with helpful suggestions. This is a journey that you are taking together, and her viewpoint is as important as yours. Point out the healthy changes your family has already made. Then, you could discuss some additional choices that she feels might work for her. Make plans to spend time together being active, such as walking a couple of laps around the mall and window shopping. Ask her to help you plan and prepare some family meals. Believe in her, that she can make changes to stay healthy and avoid some of the problems you have faced. Encourage her. If she has specific questions, suggest she accompany you on your next visit with a nutritionist.

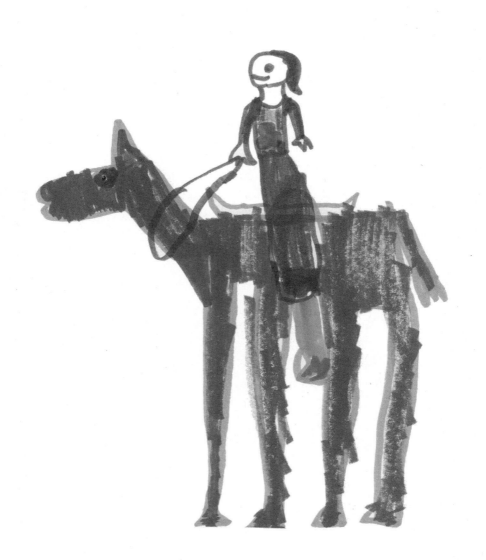

5

Pregnancy and Your Child's Growth

Kristin's parents brought her to my clinic at age 8 months. She was referred by her pediatrician for "excess weight gain." When I was reading her chart before I went in the room and saw her age, I thought it seemed odd. As I explained in the chapter about growth (Chapter 3), most babies will grow at their own rate, eating in response to their own internal cues. Why would a baby be referred for obesity?

Kristin had a birth weight of 7 pounds and now at 8 months was more than 30 pounds (the average 8-month-old weighs about 19 pounds). All babies gain weight rapidly during the first 3 to 4 months, but Kristin had taken off, shooting up at a rate that didn't follow a curve at all. Mom had breast-fed for the first 3 months but stopped after going back to work when Kristin was about 6 weeks old. Kristin had just kept eating when they switched to formula—and her weight never slowed down. The pediatrician saw them every 2 weeks, and every time her weight was up more. He suggested that they start trying to discourage her from eating too often, but she only ate every 3 to 4 hours, which is normal. She drank 2 to 3 ounces per feeding when she was 2 months and now took 5 to 6 ounces, all normal amounts. Her parents had never given her any juice, and they just started some cereal and vegetables in the last 2 months, long after her weight had gotten so high. They gave her about one jar a day—not too much.

So what is going on here? I asked Kristin's mother about the pregnancy. She said it had been very difficult. She had vomited so much that she couldn't gain weight and had been hospitalized three times for dehydration. From the beginning of the pregnancy to the end, she lost almost 25 pounds. In other words, the baby had been in a "starving" situation while inside mom. When we are losing weight, our body is forced to burn stored calories; this is called *catabolism*. When we are gaining weight or staying the same weight, our body is building and remodeling; this is called *anabolism*. In this state, supplies are plentiful for fixing broken cells and adding new layers to tissues. During the normal pattern of a single day, we go back and forth between catabolism and anabolism. Each time we eat, there is building and storing. Each time we are hungry or exercising on an empty stomach, we are burning stored calories. This pattern is normal and healthy, and probably necessary. During weight loss, burning stored calories becomes the prominent pattern.

It's very difficult to study environmental effects on pregnancy, because the effects are complicated and each woman's pregnancy has many variables. But history provides some examples. During World War II, people living in the western part of The Netherlands had their food supplies severely restricted by the Germans. This was known as the Dutch Famine. Over 6 months, the food per person was decreased to about 600 calories per day, a third of what a typical adult needs. After liberation in May 1945, food supplies returned to close to normal. Because the famine affected everyone and began and ended at the same time for the whole population, researchers were able to study what happened to babies born at different points in the famine.[16] At age 19, boys born to mothers who didn't have enough food during the first two trimesters (the first 6 months of pregnancy) were more likely to be overweight. If the mother was exposed to the famine during the later part of her pregnancy, her son was less likely to be obese. This study suggests that how well the mother eats during pregnancy has lasting effects on the baby.

It's not possible to do an experiment on pregnant mothers to learn what is best, so we have to deduce this from examples like the famine study. In a sense, Kristin experienced a famine during her development because her mom couldn't keep from vomiting all her food. Kristin's mom couldn't help it, and I hope Kristin will be fine in the long run, but her initial weight gain required attention. I think that over time, Kristin's body will figure out that it doesn't have to save all the calories coming in—that the starvation time is over and food will continue to arrive every 3 to 4 hours, no problem. The best thing for Kristin now is for her parents to plan the healthiest childhood possible. We have already talked about future plans, limiting TV for her and developing a habit of drinking water or milk if she is thirsty, rather than sweetened drinks. Her parents know that her best chance for health is to be naturally active, so they are playing games with her and letting her crawl about the living room—after having baby-proofed it, of course. They have stopped drinking sodas themselves and are working on becoming more active, so they can be the best role models possible for Kristin as she grows up.

So, would gaining a large amount of weight during pregnancy make a very skinny baby? Actually, no. Mothers who gain very large amounts of weight are also not in a healthy state, because they are constantly storing new fat. Babies born bigger than expected are called *large for gestational age.* This happens more often in mothers who have gestational diabetes during pregnancy and mothers who gain more than the recommended amount of weight during pregnancy. Children who are large for gestational age at birth and have either a mother with gestational diabetes or an overweight mother are twice as likely to be overweight and to develop diabetes by age 11 years.[17]

The activity levels of the baby can also be influenced by weight gain during pregnancy. Dr. Roberts and her colleagues studied a group of 18 infants over the first three months of life.[15] Six of the babies were from lean mothers and twelve from overweight mothers. They found that all the babies were the same as far as weight, length, amount of body fat, and metabolic rate (how they burned calories). What was different was how active they were. The babies born to lean mothers were more active. They moved around more—20% more. Does this effect continue? I don't know because the study ended at 3 months of age, and it was a small study. But the information suggests that some modeling of the "activity genes" may happen before birth.

Drs. Rising and Lifshitz studied 4-month-old babies born to overweight mothers. They found that these babies had higher body fat compared with babies from lean mothers. But also, these babies had a lower 24-hour energy expenditure rate—they burned fewer calories than the babies who had lean mothers.[18] All of these studies show the important effects that the mother's weight and habits during pregnancy can have on the baby.

Some good news is that if you are already overweight when you get pregnant, you can choose to make a difference. Dr. Davenport researched whether walking can help control the blood glucose levels of women who have gestational diabetes or who were at risk to get diabetes during pregnancy because they were overweight.[19] In her study, women exercised three to four times per week, usually beginning in the second trimester, until childbirth. This exercise, combined with healthy nutrition, helped decrease excess weight gain during the pregnancy by the mother and lessened weight retention after birth. It also helped normalize the mother's blood glucose level, which in turn kept the fetus's blood glucose in the normal range. More studies are needed to see if these changes improve the long-term growth and health of these children, but it's exciting that a simple change like regular walking during pregnancy could significantly improve your child's long-term health.

Gaining too much weight or too little weight during pregnancy can be harmful to your baby. Your obstetrician will give you a recommended weight gain based on what you weigh at the time of conception. I know that weight gain during pregnancy feels largely out of your control. But there are some simple things you can do that will help.

Tips for a Healthy Pregnancy

- After talking with your doctor, be as active as is possible for you and your baby on a daily basis. Pregnant women who are more active are less likely to have an overweight baby and pregnancy complications.[20]
- Talk with your obstetrician about your current weight and exercise habits, and make an exercise/activity plan for your pregnancy. Most pregnant women can safely walk as a form of exercise.
- This is not a time to diet or start trying to lose weight and you are not walking and exercising for weight loss. You are creating an active daily rhythm for your body that will give your baby the best start.
- Eat wholesome foods, such as locally grown vegetables, fruit, meat, eggs, and cheese and whole-grain

flours and cereals. You can choose to avoid highly processed snack and fast foods that have added sugar, fats, and preservatives. Treat yourself to the best of foods for your sake and your baby's.

◎ Drink mostly water and some milk. Limit sweetened beverages and other sources of simple sugars (including juice) and limit diet drinks. Juice can be healthy in small amounts (3–6 ounces a day).

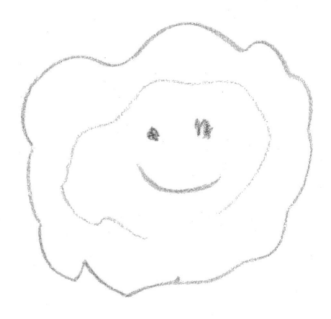

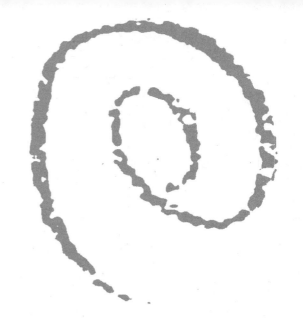

Changes for Your
Healthier Child

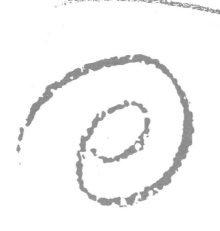

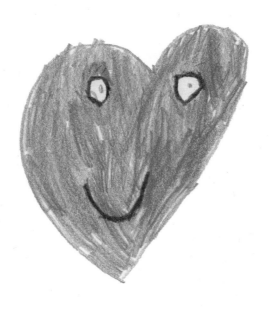

Getting Started—Together

I have met many families who want to make changes but few who know what to do. Many parents feel like my physician friend in the first chapter, whose pediatrician told her *not* to put her 6-year-old daughter on a diet . . . but *to make changes*. So, what do you change?

In this book, you will find proven methods that you can try with your own family. My hope is that you will use these tools to begin, and continue, healthy habits in your family's life.

Focus Your Effort

There is a lesson that I should tell you about first, because I have learned it the hard way: It's best to tackle one change at a time. It's tempting to ignore this advice, because often there are many things that we want to change. And in the studies of children who lost weight in a program, they usually change multiple things—the diet, the portions, the activity, the TV, and more. But making changes on your own is not a program. When parents leave my office, they go home to their busy, hectic, challenging lives. If you try to do too much at once, it can become overwhelming and you might end up not doing anything for the long term. A single change or several small changes require relatively less sacrifice and are less disturbing to other family members.

In my clinic, we make an agreement about what the parent and the child would like to work on between then and the next appointment. Sometimes, they want to do several things. I used to go along with that because I thought, "the more the better." But time and again, those families came back without having managed to make any of the changes. So, please focus your effort on one change until you have succeeded in making it part of the normal family routine. This works better than trying to change several things at once—even if your doctor wants you to change everything!

Healthy for Everyone

David was 16, a junior in high school, when he first came to see me in clinic. He was quite overweight and unhappy. His mother had discussed David's weight with his pediatrician and several specialists over the preceding years because she was worried about him. David was on several medicines. He had attention deficit disorder and gastroesophageal reflux and abdominal pain that kept him home from school several times a month. His mother was taking him back and forth to doctors on a regular basis. This was very stressful for everyone in the family. At one visit, she told me, "If I could just get David's problems settled, I could start to focus on my own health again." David's mom was also overweight and unhappy with her health. In the past, she had joined Weight Watchers and was interested in doing that again. But the time and energy for her own needs were limited because of the problems David was having.

It is very common to see families in which more than one member is overweight. The great thing is that positive changes benefit everyone. Instead of trying to solve David's problems first and then his mother's, the key for David's family was to start together in making some family changes. If you have an overweight child, don't single out your child as the target of the changes. The healthy habits described in this book are for all ages and work best when the whole family joins in. It's clear that improving physical activity and nutrition benefit everyone, no matter what their weight is.

It's a Family Change

Lydia and her parents came to see me because, at 9 years old, she had been rapidly gaining weight, and her growth chart showed she was rising well above her previous curve. Everyone in her family was chubby, but Lydia had gained enough that her mother and father felt that her problem was different from her brothers and sisters.

Lydia's pediatrician diagnosed her with high cholesterol and high triglycerides, confirming her parents' fears. In my office, Lydia saw the nutritionist first, to whom she tearfully admitted sneaking food at night and when her parents weren't around. Lydia said she felt guilty, bad, and embarrassed. She felt that her parents thought there was something wrong with her.

This is a terrible thing for a young girl to be going through. Why was she sneaking food? Well, Lydia's parents had begun limiting how much food she got. But her brothers and sisters could eat as much as they wanted, and her father continued to drink sodas as often as he liked.

Children are very sensitive to fairness and hidden messages. The restriction for Lydia meant that she was so fat (bad) that she didn't deserve seconds or sodas. One of my patients explained to me that, "at school there are lots of kids bigger than me, and they get to have seconds, but I don't" in the cafeteria at lunch. What made her so "bad" that she was being limited?

Rather than trying to *make* your child lose weight, focus on developing healthy family habits by establishing guidelines and boundaries. Restricting food and targeting one child often leads to even faster weight gain. There is more about this in Chapter 11. If you struggled with restriction in your own childhood or if you are worried that you might be restricting your child, I also encourage you to read Ellen Satter's book, *Your Child's Weight: Helping Without Harming*, about this (see Resources).

Making children feel guilty or encouraging them to eat more—both approaches interfere with their inborn way of eating. If you are watching out of the corner of your eye to see what she will eat, your child will know. If you are purposefully scooping more vegetables onto the plate of your overweight son, he will know it. "This is healthy" becomes code for, "You are fat. Eat vegetables so you won't be so fat."

You will encounter many ideas in the following chapters, some of them you can do, and some you won't need to or want to do. As you sort through your choices, here are some things to remember.

- You are the agent of change for your family. The information in this book is for parents to consider and use if it's appropriate. This is not a task for your child. Our role as parents requires us to keep growing, too.
- You will benefit from changes as much as your child will.

◎ Don't strive for perfection. Lasting change is full of ups and downs. A month will come where you don't manage to do anything, even though you wanted to. Don't sweat it. Just start that good habit up again as soon as you can.

◎ Try new things one at a time or in small amounts.

◎ If you don't get much cooperation in the family, make the new change for yourself for a while. If you sincerely enjoy the change and believe in the benefits, they'll catch on.

◎ Seek support from your spouse, a close friend, a sister or a brother. Seek support from everyone. Making changes together with another family can increase the fun, and you can support and encourage each other.

How About Your Family?

Many parents struggle with situations that interfere with their natural ability and desire to nurture their children by feeding them well. In the chapters to come, I'll share solutions that other families have used to improve their health. You may find these methods work well for you, too.

To get started, you need to think about where your family is right now. You can't make changes if you don't know what to change. The answers to the following questions will help you take a look at your current family patterns.

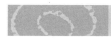

Healthy Habits Questions for Parents

Physical Activity

1. How often does your child walk or ride a bike for pleasure or necessity, such as to the grocery store, to visit a friend, or around the block?
   a. Rarely or never
   b. 2 or 3 times per week
   c. Almost every day or every day
2. How often does your child engage in physical play or activity for 20 to 30 minutes or more at a time?
   a. Rarely or never
   b. 2 to 3 times per week
   c. Almost every day or every day
3. How many hours of screen time (TV, computer, and video games) does your child have in an average day? Count weekends, too.
   a. More than 2 hours
   b. 1 to 2 hours
   c. Less than 1 hour
4. Where is the TV in your home?
   a. In the family room, the kitchen, and my child's bedroom
   b. In several rooms, but not visible from the table where we eat
   c. One TV in the main family room

Beverages

1. How many sugar-sweetened beverages does your child usually drink per day? Include soda, juice, Kool-Aid, flavored milk, sports drinks, etc. One cup (8 ounces) is 1 drink.
   a. More than 2 drinks
   b. 1 to 2 drinks
   c. Less than 1
2. How many artificially sweetened beverages (sweetened with any noncalorie sweetener) does your child usually drink per day?
   a. More than 2 drinks
   b. 1 to 2 drinks
   c. Less than 1
3. How many cups of plain water does your child usually drink per day?
   a. Less than 2 cups
   b. 2 to 3 cups
   c. 4 cups or more

(continued)

 **Healthy Habits Questions for Parents (continued)**

4. What does your child usually drink between planned meals and snacks?
    a. Sugar-sweetened beverages or artificially sweetened beverages
    b. 100% fruit juice
    c. Water
5. How many glasses of low-fat milk (2%, 1%, or fat-free) does your child usually drink per day?
    a. 0
    b. 1 glass
    c. 2 to 3 glasses

Eating

1. How many times per week does your child eat breakfast?
    a. Rarely or never
    b. 2 to 3 times per week
    c. Almost every day or every day
2. How often does your child eat at the table with one or more parents?
    a. Less than 3 times per week
    b. 3 to 5 times per week
    c. Every day
3. How often do you serve at least one vegetable with your meal?
    a. Not often
    b. 3 to 5 days per week
    c. Usually every day
4. How many times do you eat at a restaurant or bring prepared food home?
    a. Rarely or never
    b. 2 to 3 times per week
    c. 4 or more times per week
5. Where does your child usually eat meals and snacks at home?
    a. Bedroom or anywhere he or she wants
    b. Living room or family room
    c. Kitchen table, breakfast bar, or dining room table
6. How often does your child usually eat with the TV on?
    a. Most meals and snacks
    b. 3 to 4 times per week
    c. Rarely

(continued)

 **Healthy Habits Questions for Parents (continued)**

Scoring Your Quiz

Give yourself 2 points for "c" answers, 1 point for "b" answers, and 0 points for "a" answers.

If your points total	Then your family
23 or more	Has very healthy behaviors
16–22	Has habits that help prevent overweight and obesity
7–15	Is on the right track—keep making positive changes
6 or less	Has lots of room for improvement

Team Parenting

One of my patients arrived with both parents and two brothers. Ten-year-old Javon was referred to the clinic because of a rapid weight gain over the past year that was continuing, despite several visits to his pediatrician. Javon's mother had read a handout at the pediatrician's office about healthy eating and quickly listed for me the changes she had already tried to make for the family: limiting sodas, decreasing fried foods, and cooking more at home—not so much fast food. While she was talking, her husband was smiling, and the boys were giggling to each other behind their hands. With each change she listed, one of the kids would say, "But Dad still brings us soda," or "But Dad takes us out." It was clear that the kids and the dad thought that it was a great game to "outsmart mom" and still get the now unavailable items.

When I talked with the parents, it was clear that both Javon's father and mother were concerned about Javon's health. But it turned out that the children were regularly sneaking sodas from dad's hidden supply, which he hadn't been willing to give up. Having sodas in the house felt like a big problem to Javon's mom. But this wasn't the only challenge. The central issue was the lack of agreement between the parents, and the kids were using it to their advantage.

Although Javon's father agreed with the food changes in principle, he had not committed to them for himself. Parents often differ on the level of control, permissiveness, timing, and arrangement in feeding children. During our talk, Javon's father came to see that the small changes his wife was trying to make were an important way to care for his son. It was only then that he was ready to make changes. He agreed to stop supplying the sodas that undermined his wife's plan for improvement. Everyone in the family, including the dad, switched from drinking soda to mostly drinking water instead, a simple but powerful healthy habit. With his father and mother as positive role models, in two months' time, Javon's rapid weight gain had stopped, and he was again following his own natural growth curve. He changed from gaining 10 pounds a month to a stable growth pattern—a wonderful achievement.

Conflicts can sometimes arise because your spouse or partner has a very different approach to feeding your children. What happened in Javon's family shows why parents need to agree on how to feed children and be supportive of each other. It took the viewpoint of someone outside the family for the father to understand why these changes were so important. Once the family worked in harmony, those changes were possible.

Forget the Bathroom Scale

Some professionals who work with overweight children (and adults) ask them to weigh in every day. This is one way to check whether changes are being made. I discourage this, although it's true that monitoring has its benefits. For example, when you are driving and see a police officer with a radar gun pointed at you, you slow down and quickly glance at the speedometer. Knowing that someone else is watching your behavior supports good behavior. But your child's weight is not a behavior. It's only a number that is the result of many complex influences—genetics plus years of family habits and individual things that you do, they do, and our society does.

So, in my work with overweight children, I like to monitor *behaviors* not weight. I want to know how many times you played outside in the past week and how many glasses of water you drank instead of drinking something with sugar in it. In my experience, the weight usually comes down on its own—slowly and surely—when healthy changes are made. If you are worried about your son's weight, take him for a walk to the park this weekend or go ride bikes together, but don't put him on the bathroom scale. That can feel like failing a test, which doesn't feel good to anyone.

I don't recommend putting your child on the scale to check up on him or her. Most of the kids in my clinic notice that their pants starts to feel a little looser long before the scale responds.

Focus on Healthy Family Habits

Simple lifestyle changes like the ones we cover in this book can slow down or reverse a trend toward obesity. If you are starting early, it will be easier. Your child is still growing taller and has a flexible metabolism (see Chapter 4). And some parents find it's easier to try positive lifestyle changes while their children are young. The old saying rings true: An ounce of prevention is worth a pound of cure.

Please don't use your child's weight or BMI as a marker of short-term progress. Your child's weight is something that in many ways you and your child *don't* have control over. Instead, pay attention to the factors you can control. You can decide to take your child outside to play instead of watching TV. You can provide drinking water at home instead of sodas. You control which cereals are in your pantry and can choose high-fiber, low-sugar ones to offer your children. But you don't get to decide what your child weighs. A lifetime of health depends more on the healthy habits you are building day by day than on your child's current BMI.

Simple Changes to Consider

Making changes always takes time. In the following chapters, you will read about lots of changes to consider. Remember:

choose one change at a time to focus on. As you succeed, and one change becomes a family habit, you can build on that foundation by choosing another change to make.

- Spend time playing outside each day.
- Limit television and computer screen time to 1 hour per day, excluding homework.
- Drink more water.
- Prepare and eat breakfast and dinner at home.
- Eat meals together.
- Serve more vegetables every day.
- Make mealtime a pleasant and nurturing experience.
- Let your children choose how much they will eat of the foods you serve them.

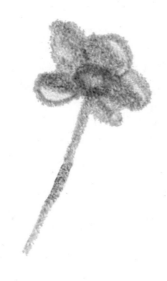

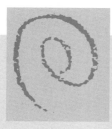

Question for the Psychologist

Q **All this change is going to be hard for my 10-year-old. How do I get him to understand the importance?**

A Don't expect your ten-year-old to understand. As the parent, you must find out what is best and apply this to the family. Your child's task is to cooperate and to learn from you. You are wise to realize that your son will resist the changes; no one likes to change. I suggest you start by having a brief discussion with him about the changes and why they are necessary for the health of the entire family, including for you. Listen to his objections, give him sympathy, and ask him for suggestions on how the changes might be made easier for him. Then stick to your plan. It is best to avoid arguing; don't try to defend your decision or to persuade him. You cannot *make* him cooperate. Invite him to cooperate and then use rewards for cooperation and negative consequences for lack of cooperation. For example, if your son desires computer or video time, you can limit it as a consequence and provide it (in small amounts) as a reward. Pretty soon, he will cooperate. Kids will test you to see if you are serious. You should expect to have to apply a negative consequence or two before you get cooperation. You will be surprised how soon the resistance will be over.

7

Raising an Active Child

Philip was 12 years old and overweight. He already had several complications of weight gain, including high blood pressure and fatty liver disease. As we walked through the hallways to the Emory Clinic where the research MRI was located, his little brother ran ahead and behind and ahead again, in the typical manner of an energetic 3-year-old. I noticed that Philip was starting to breathe hard and so was his mother. I slowed down and we kept going, but both of them were sweating and breathing hard when we arrived at the end of the hallway.

Unfortunately, this is not an isolated event. By the time children come to see me, most of them have a hard time walking the equivalent of two city blocks. I asked Philip and his mother to start taking daily walks. The first trip might be to the corner and back. The key for them was to do a small amount every day and add distance as it became easier.

Start Early

What I found most striking was that the 3-year-old was running circles around the other two family members. If you start early and capitalize on the natural energy your children have, it will be much easier to keep them going into adulthood. So what can you do?

- Start early.
- Get creative about adding daily activity into your and your child's lives.
- Walk with the stroller or carry your baby.
- When they are toddlers, let children walk a block or two and then ride in the stroller if they get tired. Don't keep them in the stroller the whole time.
- When they get a little older, they can ride a tricycle, scooter, or bike alongside as you walk.
- By the time they are about 5 years old, most kids should be able to walk 1 to 2 miles with a little practice— and even farther if you walk or hike regularly.

Babies at Play

One of my friends at work told me she didn't like "babies in a bucket." I didn't understand at first—but she was talking about how some babies spend most of their time in a chair, swing, or stroller. She wanted her babies to be out on the carpet or in their playpen scooting around and crawling and pulling up. Most babies are naturally active, and their play time out in the open is important. It is almost impossible for scientists to study the

Need Some Reasons to Limit Screen Time?

Dr. Zimmerman and colleagues tested children younger than 3 years old and found that, as hours spent watching TV per day went up, the worse the kids did on a memory test, a reading comprehension test, and a reading recognition test.[21]

These same researchers also showed that children 2 to 5 years old are 34% more likely to be overweight if they watch 2 or more hours of TV per day. Any computer time at all in this age group also made the child more likely to be overweight.[22]

Bottom line: Screen time isn't healthy for young children.

If you find this surprising, you aren't alone. In the United States, 90% of 2-year-olds regularly watch some sort of media, despite the recommendations of the American Association of Pediatrics that they not watch any.[23] It's time to start a new trend!

effects of things like this—so I'm going with my friend's maternal instincts, which I am sure are right on track. She points out that babies and little children are often "parked" in front of the TV, again decreasing their natural instincts to play and move around. The American Academy of Pediatrics recommends *no TV before age 2 years*.[23] This is valuable time for you to play with and talk and read to your baby. The TV cannot replace you!

Make a Commitment, Make It a Habit

My neighbors, T and R, take their two kids to the park every night after dinner unless it is pouring down rain. I asked T how she makes it work for her family.

"We just do it," she said. "It's what we do after dinner, every day, whether they want to or not. It's part of our evening ritual. Now they just expect it. Making an incentive is good, too, such as getting to ride their scooter or bike there and back or having a family kickball game when we get there. The kids also love it when dad plays 'monster' and chases them around the playground."

In my neighborhood, we are lucky because there is a park at the end of our street, and many families play there on the weekends and afternoons and evenings. T is exactly right about what gets you to the park—commitment and habit. If there is no park nearby, try a family stroll after dinner. Depending on their ages, the kids can ride a bike or tricycle while you walk or ride a skate board or skate. Don't use motorized or battery-operated vehicles. You want their muscles to get the benefit—and remember the protective helmets.

My colleague Jennifer suggests that if you can't make it to the park before or after dinner, turn on some music and dance. That gets your bodies moving and your blood flowing. You might get a DVD of country line dancing or a samba class and have fun learning new steps together. She says, "Turn on the music and dance! But don't forget to close the blinds first, so you are free to move without worrying about how you look. I am a terrible dancer, so my girls did a lot of laughing while we danced. Rather than be offended, I played the comic role and created even sillier dances. We danced and laughed until we fell on the floor! Kids love participating in physical activities with their parents—even the 12-year-olds who seem to always roll their eyes at you. Your child will be more active if you are actively engaged with him or her. Don't worry if you don't have certain skills. Teach your kids that you don't have to be good at something to enjoy it. The more laughter, the better."

No Time to Play

When Ashley first came to our clinic, her mother was visibly upset. Her mom clearly had struggled with her own weight and was worried because Ashley "just kept getting bigger." At 8 years old, she was "the biggest in the class." She had started to play soccer but quit because she felt out of place with the smaller girls, and she was so much slower.

We talked about many issues at the first appointment, but one thing was clear—their daily schedule was challenging.

Ashley's mother drove her to a special school with a top reputation for math and science, about a 50-minute drive in typical rush hour traffic. Then her mother drove another 45 minutes to work. Because they left so early, breakfast was eaten in the car, if at all. Ashley's school had physical education classes, but the teachers were worried about Ashley getting tired, so they let her sit down often. Ashley had gotten the "hint," so she would ask to sit down so she wouldn't always be the last in every game. She went to an after-school program until her mom arrived at 5:30 p.m. They got home around 6:30, often picking up something for dinner on the way home, ate a quick dinner, and then started on the homework—at least an hour's worth. Then it was off to bed to start the whole routine again.

Because of the schedule during the week, Ashley and her mother got no physical activity and had little quality meal time together. Dinner was something to get done—and was often rushed because of the pressure to get her homework finished.

I admit that the first thing that came to my mind was, "Take Ashley out of the private school and simplify your life—it's only second grade!" However, that isn't what I said. Every family has their own set of responsibilities and challenges. I admire parents like Ashley's mother. The sacrifices she is making with such love are amazing gifts to Ashley. But something needed to change—Ashley's health was suffering. So, where to make some adjustments? I have discussed this issue with many families, and I think it's best to identify each family's "low-hanging fruit." These are the one or two changes that, given your family and your schedules, won't be as hard to reach as the others. Start with something that is possible for you and see how it goes.

Ashley's mom wanted to make changes and decided to begin by focusing on getting more physical activity. It turned out that Ashley's after-school program offered some active classes. Ashley could join fencing or karate instead of sitting in a classroom doing school work. And, although it seemed like there was no extra time in the evening, her mom agreed that Ashley could play outside in the backyard, instead of watching TV, while her mother got dinner ready. There was flexible time on the weekends, too, for playing outside and going on hikes in a park with a 4-mile walking path. Ashley's mom wanted to exercise as well. She could walk while Ashley biked along with her. They both tried walking the path, but Ashley didn't like it—despite the fact that her mom tried to make it fun by chatting and playing word games. So they decided to try it again, with Ashley biking instead.

The bottom line is that kids need regular, active play to be part of their daily lives. Really, adults do too. It was great that Ashley's mom had tried walking with her on the weekends, but the 4 miles with no other activity might have been a bit much for Ashley. Also, instead of walking the same path each week, her mom could add variety with other outdoor activities like swimming or canoeing or hiking. She could let Ashley choose an activity for one weekend a month to help Ashley "buy in." They could invite one of Ashley's friends to come along.

Two busy parents I know take their kids to the YMCA every Sunday afternoon. The kids spend an hour playing in child care while both parents work out, and then they all go to the pool for an hour to play. Another family usually arrives at the same time, and the kids now look forward to playing together each week.

Busy schedules make it harder to have a naturally active child. And the activities themselves, like soccer practice and ballet, can make you even busier. So where do you get the time? One good place to take back your precious time is from "screen time."

Reducing TV: Tips from Parents

The current recommendation is to limit TV or screen time (video games, etc.) to 1 hour per day for children age 2 and up. But the fact is that children of all ages spend more time in front of a TV or video game than ever before. I commonly hear estimates of 3 to 4 hours on school nights and much more on weekends. Almost all American households now have a television, and many have TVs in several rooms, including the child's bedroom. In fact, more than half of all children ages 8 to 18 have a TV in their bedrooms.[24] So, whenever I meet parents who have successfully controlled the time spent in front of the TV, I am impressed and try to learn how they did it. Here are some of their tips for you.

- Start early by keeping the TV limited from the beginning. It helps not to have more than one TV in the house. Remember, no TV at all before age 2 is the recommendation.
- Don't get cable for your kids. It presents too many choices.
- Use DVDs. There are no commercials, and you can control the content. "I pop a 30-minute cartoon in every afternoon at 5:30. They get to calm down while I get things together for dinner. They know that it is all they get—just one DVD a day."
- Let them dance along with music or with a dance class DVD.
- Try a "no TV" week. Get the whole family to participate and rediscover board games, cards, dancing, playing outside, and talking.
- Buy a TV monitor. These devices are an excellent way to manage TV time. For about $90, you can purchase a small monitor that controls the power to the TV, computer, or video game. Time can be added on a daily, weekly, or monthly basis. Every time your child watches, they are "using up" their minutes. When the minutes are gone, the TV turns off. It reduces arguing and can help control access if you can't be home all the time. (See Resources for an example.)

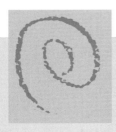

Question for the Psychologist

Q **We put TVs and computers in all the kids' rooms years ago. Now I want to take them out. How do I make it not seem like a punishment for being fat?**

A Good for you that you want to reestablish the bedroom as a sleeping room instead of an individual living room. This promotes good sleep habits and can also bring the disconnected family back together. There is no need for a child's weight to be a factor in this good decision. Tell them that you did not realize how much healthier it is not to have TVs in the bedrooms and that you did not realize how separate all of you would become when you each watch your own TV. Find a quiet place other than the bedroom for the computer.

"Active" Video Games?

Dr. Steve Reichman, an exercise physiologist at Texas A&M University, bought one of the new video games that promote being active for his own kids. When I asked him what he thought about it, he said to watch out. It turns out that only some of the games are actually active. Some are just hand movements, no "big muscle" moving. The other challenge is that the amount of exercise depends on the personality of the person playing. One of his sons is wild when playing the tennis game—running back and forth and swinging his arms. His son's friend was swinging, too, but quickly figured out that he could sit on the couch and just move his hand and wrist. If your child is naturally very active, the game will build on that. If you have a naturally inactive child, you might want to "test" the game before owning it.

Overall, these new video games seem to be more active than the older video games but certainly are less active than

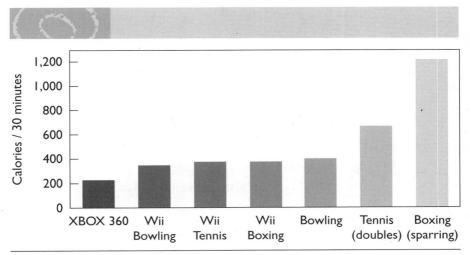

Source: Adapted from Reference 25.

actually playing the sport. Dr. Graves and his colleagues studied 11 children playing different active computer games and measured how many calories they burned over time compared to the real sport.[25] Of the sports they tested, real boxing burned the most and the XBOX360 games burned the fewest.

Your Child Can Play Outside—Even in the Rain

What do your children do instead of watching TV? They can go outside and play. I suggest that you set an expectation that they will play outside for a certain amount of time, usually 45 to 60 minutes—less if younger or if you have concerns about their safety. If it's cold, put a coat and hat on them. If it's raining, they can play with an umbrella and boots. Playing outside every day is good for them. It doesn't have to take a lot of time. If you need 10 minutes to get something done, send your child outside to play for 10 minutes.

It is not your responsibility to provide constant entertainment. Children need to learn to entertain themselves. Almost any outdoor activity will be more active than sitting on the couch or in front of a screen. If you look out the win-

dow and your son or daughter is sitting on the ground looking for a four leaf clover, don't worry about it. It is great that
he or she is self-entertaining and outside. Nature is good for
us all, but children don't operate like adults with regard to
getting active. We do more deliberate, focused exercise, like
walking a certain distance every day. Children are better
off with low-key, low-pressure playing, especially younger
children.

Although they don't need your constant companionship,
it is good to play with your children sometimes. One of my
patients told me, "Please tell my mom to play with us." His
mom laughed and, I think, blushed a little. Her son wanted
her to come out in the backyard and play with him, but she
felt too busy. I could see how much it meant to him. As a busy
professional, I understand that a working mom can't be in the
backyard every day instead of making dinner. So we compro-
mised. His mom agreed to come outside once or twice a week,
and he agreed to play on his own the other days.

If your neighborhood isn't safe, try taking turns with
another mother or father to watch both sets of kids or take them
to a safe park to play once or twice a week. Enlist older children
to help watch younger children. Have a neighborhood kickball
game or block picnic in the summer so you can get to know the
other parents on your street. Start a neighborhood play group
every Saturday afternoon where you get to meet with other parents and the kids can play—in the street or a yard.

Ways to Be More Active

I recently heard the neighbor kids playing in their back yard
in a new pile of sand. "Where did you get the sand?" I asked.
"Santa!" they said. What a great Christmas gift. Their dad is
building a new wooden sandbox to go around the new sand.
A pile of soft clean sand is a great enticement to play outside.
(If there are cats in the neighborhood, cover the sand with a
tarp at night.) Here are more tips for inviting your children to
be active.

- Install a play set in the back yard.
- Buy balls, bats, jump-ropes, and Frisbees for birthday and Christmas gifts and help your children learn to use them.
- Put up a basketball hoop (at a lower height for the little girls and boys).
- Try a "no cords, no batteries" policy for birthday parties when other people bring gifts.
- Have active "play dates" with other families: meet at the park or YMCA or local pool instead of places to eat.
- Turn on music in the family area at home . . . instead of the TV.
- Exercise through everyday activity: vacuuming, sweeping the porch, carrying the laundry up and down stairs, taking the garbage out. Your children benefit from sharing the responsibility to help maintain their home, too.
- Rake the leaves together (don't use the blower).

Think About Where You Live

If you are moving, think about how your choice will affect your family's physical activity level. Is there a park? Are there bike lanes? Can your child walk to school? Is there a community center nearby? I live in the sprawling city of Atlanta where people think nothing of a 1-hour commute. I chose a smaller house that is 8 minutes by bike and 8 minutes by car from my work. A couple of times a week, I walk or bike the hilly 1½ miles to work. Because I don't have to use the parking garage when I bike, I actually get to my office faster. I pass many children walking to our neighborhood elementary school, and I wave to the crossing guard as I make the turn every morning.

I know that, as a parent, you make many hard choices, but please put this one in the equation. *Walking to school for a few years may be right up there with how good the test scores are as far as the lifelong benefit to your child.*

Have you considered having just one car? This is a suggestion from my sister. You naturally end up walking and biking more because sometimes you don't have the car available. It also saves money and gas.

It may seem surprising, but children who live in "the country" are more likely to be overweight than city children. When I talk to my patients from rural areas, it is clear that one of the reasons is low activity levels.

Billy's parents told me that, "He goes down to the creek all the time." He was in my office for high liver enzymes and a long history of being overweight. As we tried to sort through his risk factors, we talked about his diet, activities, and habits. I was encouraged when I heard that he was playing outside and asked how far it was to the creek. It was about half a mile, and he went almost every afternoon to play. Unfortunately, a year earlier his parents had bought him a 4-wheeler that he was riding to the creek. So, although he was playing outside, his activity level had decreased a lot after this gift. I think that gift contributed to his new fatty liver disease. His body really needed that 1-mile walk every day.

Let Kids Move Themselves (No Engines)

Another person I know, who lives in a rural area, told me that his kids all have go-carts and 4-wheelers. He was happy with how much they liked being outside. Unfortunately, he is very overweight, and so I know that his children have an increased risk of weight problems. While I appreciate that these vehicles can be fun, I would have suggested that he steer away from anything with a motor or battery power while his children are in the growing years. Children need to exert themselves, and pushing along on a bike, skateboard, or skates or their own two feet is what they need.

One of my patients is a 12-year-old born with cerebral palsy. He can't walk, and his right hand works much better than his left. Because he can't use his hands well, he was given a motorized wheelchair. When he is in his room, his parents

The Exercise–School Performance Connection

Regular exercise can help your overweight child perform better in school. Dr. Davis studied 90 overweight children.[26] Some of them agreed to exercise 40 minutes 5 times per week. When tested at the end of the study, the children who exercised improved their "executive functioning." These tasks include the ability to plan, organize, perform goal-directed activities, think creatively, and self-regulate thoughts. All of these tasks are critical to not only doing well in school but daily living as well!

and brother bring him what he needs, including his food, because that is easier. He had been in physical therapy, but that ended after they moved and his insurance changed. After the move, his weight started to go up dramatically, and he gained more than 20 pounds in 6 months. His neurologist referred him to me. His parents were very worried and wanted to help him.

We came up with a plan to start increasing his activity level. He could propel himself around the house instead of using the motor. He rolled himself to the dinner table and started using his ramp again for the exercises that he used to do. His face got slimmer, and he stabilized his weight. A year later, he weighs exactly the same as he did last year, but he has grown in height, so he's slimming down. I hope he will be able to get a special wheelchair that works for one-handed turning so he can propel himself outside the house, too. Getting outside under your own power is a goal for everyone I see!

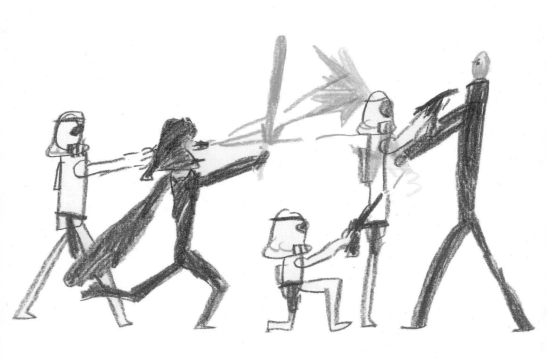

Raising an Active Teen

*J*ose was 17 years old when he first came to see me. He had been gaining weight rapidly for years and had reached 275 pounds along with having high blood pressure and type 2 diabetes. On the plus side, he was a charming, engaging young man, had a good social life, and did well in school. He and his mom drove to all activities. There was a shopping center near their house, and Jose used to play basketball with friends at a local hoop but hadn't played recently. By the end of our visit, Jose had chosen "walking more" as a positive change to work on. Six weeks later at the return visit, I wanted to find out how it went. At this time, Atlanta was in the middle of an extreme drought; there had been no rain for 6 months. The lack of rain was in the headlines and on the news almost every day. "So, how did your plan to walk more go?" I asked. He shook his head a little. "I didn't do it as much as I planned." I asked what happened, and he replied, "I wanted to walk more, but it rained." And then we all started laughing. He realized as soon as he said it how silly it sounded, and it certainly tickled his mom and me.

Now, I am sure that one of the times Jose set out to go for a walk, it did rain. We have lots of little isolated showers in the summer, so one neighborhood gets a quick downpour while the rest of the city is dry. What this really meant, though, was that Jose was not ready to make a change.

I did not get upset with Jose. I didn't try to make him feel guilty. I accepted that he wasn't ready to make the change, and we spent some time problem-solving to see what else he could do. At the next appointment, Jose had big news. He had started walking! He was walking to the local shopping center several times a week; it was about a mile in each direction. He had also started playing basketball with his friends on a regular basis. He was proud of his achievements. No matter what, having regular physical activity will be healthier for him both physically and emotionally.

It's important to give children, especially teenagers, some room to develop their own motivations. Jose was probably testing me. If he didn't walk, was I going to reject him or tell him he was a bad person for not doing the thing that he so much needs to do? A lot of parents tell me that their child "never uses the treadmill that I bought." The child probably didn't want it in the first place. The treadmill was bought because there is something "wrong" with the child. It's a constant reminder that someone thinks he or she is too fat and needs to be on it while their friends play or watch TV.

I know that, unfortunately, a lot of misguided advice comes from the medical community. When I am speaking, I ask physicians in the audience not to prescribe time on an exercise machine for children and teenagers (treadmills seem to be the most popular). This type of exercise routine might work for an adult, who can be motivated by the positive effects they feel afterward and disregard the discomfort they feel while doing the exercise. Many adults even start to enjoy increasing the abilities of their muscles and take pleasure in the activity. Children, including teenagers, are better off doing naturally active things and social physical activity. They enjoy or are motivated by those kinds of activities and not by a desire to lose weight or their doctor's desire for them to lose weight. Treadmills are for adults. Playing is for children and teens.

Your child needs daily opportunities to use his or her muscles. This is the way nature intended it. There is a bonus for having and using muscles. Muscles burn three times as many calories as fat does. Muscles even burn calories when the body is at rest.

The Double Standard

Recently, a new patient came in with her father. She was an attractive young lady who appeared older than her 11 years. She had been referred by another doctor, a specialist who had been seeing her for several years but "hadn't gotten anywhere" with her weight-related high blood pressure. When I entered the room, it was clear that there were emotional issues. The young lady wouldn't make eye contact with me, and dad seemed upset, too. He explained that his daughter was clearly fat and wouldn't cooperate with using the treadmill. He had offered to pay her. He had it set up right in front of the TV— and yet, if she did use it, which was rarely, she put it on the lowest setting and barely moved.

Dad was overweight as well and emphasized that he required six pills a day for his hypertension, high cholesterol, and type 2 diabetes. But did he use the treadmill? "No, of course not!" was his answer to me. When I asked him how his two children (the 13-year-old son was overweight, too)

Strength Training in Children and Teens

- There is no set age at which children may start. They do need to be able to accept and follow instructions.
- It's best for your child to be in programs with other children close to their own age.
- The social aspect of a program is the most important part for a child or teen.
- Avoid highly competitive programs. Instead, look for programs that encourage self-improvement and individual accomplishments.
- Free weights, medicine balls, and rubber tubing are all great for kids.
- Look for instructors who emphasize acquiring new skills and practicing good sportsmanship, self-discipline, responsibility, self-esteem, and leadership.
- Pay attention to pain. Pain during an exercise means stop. Pain after an exercise means skip that exercise during the next session. Pain after 2 days means that the injury may need medical evaluation.

Source: Reference 27.

could get more exercise, he said they could walk up and down the big hill in front of their house. I asked if he ever walked the hill—again, an emphatic "no."

Whether she can explain it or not, his daughter clearly sees the incongruity here: that her father has three weight-related diseases and is more overweight than she, yet he doesn't do any of the exercise that he is asking her to do. It's a double standard. In the end, a child of this age is more likely to *do as you do,* not as you say.

Getting the Whole Family in the Game

One good way to take the pressure off your child and to increase the activity level for the whole family is to participate in a sport or a community event together. For example, think about a 5 K (3-mile) walk/run for the whole family. If you haven't been walking at all, plan for at least 8 weeks of preparation time for a 5 K or try a 1-mile fun walk. Start with walking for 15 or 20 minutes and increase gradually. If you do too much the first time out and everyone is sore the next day, you are not likely to get your child to participate happily again. Try to walk at least two times a week. The best schedule is to go out every other day when you are learning a new activity. For running, look online or in a running magazine for a training guide and helpful suggestions on how to build up to a new running goal. Look for local running clubs or organizations that teach people to start running. For bike riding, many bike stores have organized rides and will help you and your child learn to bike safely as well. (Don't forget a helmet for everyone!)

Establishing a routine is a good way to keep an activity going. Decide on the time it's going to happen and do it, for example, every Saturday morning or every Tuesday night. I run every other day. I don't have to think about whether I feel like running. On the way home from work when I am tired, I think about whether I ran the day before. If I did, then I walk or stretch and do yoga. If I didn't, I go running. The routine makes it easy. And I always feel better after exercise. It's interesting that you can be so tired before exercising, and after exercising, have more energy than you've had all day.

Another motivator is having an event to prepare for. If your son or daughter knows that the family 5 K walk is coming up next month, he or she will be more motivated to get out there. I have started a "wall of honor," a big bulletin board where I post the pictures of my patients making big achievements. If your child or your family finishes a 5 K walk or run, hikes to the top of a mountain, or bikes across the state, put a picture on your refrigerator, or start your own "wall of success" at home so you can all see and celebrate the great things your child has done.

If you need new ideas and motivation, subscribe to a magazine about active living like *Outside* or *Running*—or go to the library to read the magazines there and check out books on sports or activities that interest you. Take classes, be curious, ask questions, and keep learning. This is so much better for all of you than sitting on the couch and watching other people do things. You are now living your own lives—and hopefully, having some fun, too.

Sports and Organized Activities

My sister lives near a neighborhood with a community center but she doesn't actually live in that neighborhood. She submitted a special request to enroll her children in dance and soccer classes there because they are a one-car family and she wanted to be able to bike over with the kids. Not only did she get in, but she was given the classes she asked for, making her schedule much easier. Take the first step—make a call. Visit the center nearest you and see what they have for your children. Many communities are starting to provide skate parks for kids. Explore and see what your area offers. Ask for what you need; the worst that can happen is that they say "no."

- Start a sport or activity through a local community center or YMCA or YWCA. There are lots of programs for children.
- Don't start too many new activities at once, or you can make yourselves crazy.
- Choose activities your child finds interesting.
- Biking or walking to the activity is great.

Give It Time

Don't give up on a new activity if the kids (or you) don't like it the first few times. Children will resist doing something that is unfamiliar; actually, we all do. Nobody likes feeling awkward, so help them through that phase. You can't like what you don't know. Make a plan and stick to it. For example, if your child signs up for the summer soccer league, he should finish even if it doesn't seem as much fun as he expected. Especially for younger kids, don't expect them to want to play

Strong Body, Strong Spirit

It's common for girls who want to lose weight or look thinner to start running or going to the gym. However, activities such as yoga and Pilates have a big advantage over other approaches. These exercises teach you to become aware of your own body and breath. It's an internal thing and works on getting you to accept yourself and opening gently to become stronger and more flexible. It's not just your body that becomes stronger, it's your spirit. You accomplish something—like a handstand. Girls in my class who do a handstand for the first time are so excited. There are benefits outside of class, too. They become more connected to their bodies, so they start to think about what they are putting into their bodies and making better choices about what to drink and eat.

—Catherine Graber, Personal Trainer, Yoga and Pilates Instructor

every time. Don't get upset or put pressure on them to perform. It's fine to sit on the sideline and watch on a day they don't feel like playing. At the end of the summer, decide together if he or she wants to sign up for the next session. If not, choose something else. Your child is gaining experience in different areas and that is valuable.

Leagues and sports for children have gotten quite sophisticated and very competitive in many communities. This is good and bad. It means that those children with talent in sports have more opportunity, but it also makes it harder for the average kid to stay active in sports. Look to your YMCA or less competitive leagues if your child is sitting on the bench a lot or is feeling bad about not keeping up. Talk about what it means to do something for fun, not for winning. And try to keep your own competitive nature out of the arena.

Body Weight Pressures in Sports

I have counseled many a young man not to gain more weight for football. The pressure to do that is not always spoken aloud. I often meet teens and young adults who gained weight for a sport and later suffered health problems because the weight stayed on after the sport ended. There are other sports, such as wrestling, ballet, and gymnastics, where maintaining a very low weight is valued. My colleague, now a dietitian, was a highly skilled gymnast and remembers fasting and dehydrating so she could "make weight" at practice. These pressures are so damaging to young bodies, minds, and hearts. Weight loss practices like these can delay or stop normal physical development and lead to eating disorders, increased infections, and depression. Excess weight gain in athletes can lead to all the diseases listed in Chapter 2 if the fitness level drops in later life.

Young people, coaches, and parents need to know that physique does not affect performance. In other words, a very talented athlete may be chubby or thin, tall or short. So, how do you help your child navigate the pressures to gain or to lose weight? Here are some practical recommendations to help you protect your child.[28]

- Except in sports that require a weigh-in, coaches should not discuss weight or weight loss with an athlete.
- Many coaches do not have the nutrition background to do weight counseling and may not understand the difference between weight and body fitness and performance.
- Athletes involved in a sport with required weigh-ins should compete at a weight that is appropriate for their height and body shape and use good practices for weigh-ins—no vomiting or dehydration.
- For wrestling, mat-side weigh-ins will help decrease the practice of dehydrating for weigh-ins that occur in advance of the match.
- Female athletes should eat enough calories to meet their energy requirements and have their menses (periods). If her periods stop, your daughter needs to

see her pediatrician, decrease training, and increase calories and nutrients in her diet.

- The BMI for an athlete can be misleading. Muscle mass weighs a lot, so the BMI may appear "too high."
- In sports where weight gain is valued, remind your young athlete and the coach that improper gain can lead to slower speed and decreased agility and endurance.
- Talk about and discourage the use of supplements for athletic performance. Few if any are tested in children, and in my opinion, none of them are better than a good-quality, balanced diet with plenty of protein, fat, whole-grain carbohydrates, vegetables, and fruits. Some supplements can be harmful; for example, high doses of creatine (a protein product taken to increase short-term muscle performance) can harm the kidneys.
- Help your child understand the limits of genetics. Some people make bulky muscles and some make long, thin ones. It's hard to change your body shape much by working out and eating or not eating. It's healthier to learn to enjoy a well-trained body than to focus on how it looks.
- Eating more calories can be combined with doing more strength training to encourage muscle growth instead of growth of fat deposits.
- Weight gain for a sport should be gradual, about 1% of total body weight per week.

Sibling Rivalry

Within families, different children excel in different areas. You can help your child with finding his or her own identity and space to achieve. Jerrod was overweight and clearly not happy to be in my office. He told me that he was trying to be more active, but his mother also explained that, "His brother is the athletic one." His older brother was 16 and Jerrod was 14, and I could see that the natural competition of brothers was making it hard for him to feel good about his own activity. No matter what he did, he always seemed to be less good at it than his brother. If you have an athletic child who excels on the basketball team, think about enrolling your next child in something completely different like swimming or soccer or volleyball. Each child can be "the best" in your family at their own sport.

Jerrod ended up joining the high school band that summer. Camp was physically challenging, with all-day marching in the heat carrying his instrument. He got stronger, and 6 months later when he came back, his jeans were loose and he was visibly leaner and more confident. It was such a pleasure to hear him explain that he felt stronger and that he was proud of what he could do with his strong body.

Plan Active Vacations

When I was growing up, most of our vacations involved camping . . . in the Grand Canyon, Bryce Canyon, or on the mosquito-ridden banks of the Platt River. We camped all over Kentucky, my home state. The main event on most days was a hike up one of the trails or taking a walk with the rangers to learn about the local plants and wildlife.

Although camping is not for every family, hiking and visiting national or state parks has many benefits for children. They learn about the environment and to appreciate the wonders around them. They also get to run up the trails to get ahead of you and use their healthy bodies to explore.

Vacations are a great time to be more active. If you go to the beach, walk up the beach for a mile or two with your children to see what you can find. If you visit relatives, plan an excursion together to a nearby state or city park. If you go to a new city—walk from the hotel to the restaurant or to the museum instead of taking a taxi or car.

Food on Vacation

Plan ahead. Find out if the hotel has rooms with a refrigerator or kitchenette. I do a lot of traveling for work, and one trick I have learned is to plan my breakfast. I pack a bag or box of cereal and, after I arrive, buy milk to put in the little refrigerator in my room. Then I can have a filling bowl of healthy cereal each morning and not deal with the hotel breakfast buffet.

Renting your own cabin or condo gives you more control over your food than being in a hotel room. If you have a kitchen, it's much easier to plan and sit down for breakfast and dinner and pack lunches. You can enjoy some dinners out but not be the captive of the restaurant industry for all your meals. I also find this to be much cheaper than eating out three meals each day.

- Bring your own cereal and snacks on trips.
- Pack sandwiches and water for car trips, which limits the need to stop somewhere and buy something.
- In the car, it's easy to be bored. Don't use snacks as entertainment.

The Bottom Line

Playing, vacationing, and eating together are things that healthy families do. I encourage you to enjoy this time that you have together. Use it in ways that make you feel more alive and that will create family pride and treasured memories.

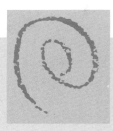

Question for the Psychologist

Q **Even though I know I shouldn't, I still wish my teenage daughter was thin. I know what she is going to go through if she
stays heavy. How do I truly accept her as she is and stop secretly
pushing for thinner?**

A It is natural for you to wish "thinness" for your daughter. Good parents
want what is best for their child, including a healthy weight. But you are
right: the first step is to accept your daughter as she is right now. She will feel it
even if your "pushing" is silent. She needs your acceptance to feel good about
herself. Also, she needs the space to decide for herself what she wants to do
without having to prove her independence by reacting against your wishes.

Our culture and media push young girls to consider images of beauty that
may be extreme and too low in weight to be healthy. And in movies and television there is always an overweight character, jolly but at the receiving end of
jokes and teasing, too. That's a confusing message for our children. What are
your feelings about heavy people? Did you know that in the past, and in some
cultures now, a round body is considered beautiful? Your daughter is unique on
the face of this Earth and has many qualities to admire—maybe she is good-
natured or a whiz at math, or has a keen interest in a hobby or playing a musi-
cal instrument. Be glad for every aspect of her life that is healthy, and enjoy her
as she is. Trust her to cope with what her future brings. When you decide to
make some changes for your family, don't make them just to help her look thinner, make them to help each of you become healthier in the bodies that you
already have. In this way, you can love and accept your daughter just as she is
while choosing habits that you know will benefit her health—and your own.

9

Getting Enough Rest

Sleep is important for healthy active bodies. Studies show that children who are overweight get less sleep. I am not sure which one comes first, the weight problem or the sleep problem, but getting enough sleep is important for children in many ways.

Growing happens while you are sleeping. Sleep improves daytime functioning and energy levels. This is the basic stuff. But in my clinic, I find that many families have forgotten to pay attention to sleep. Older children (teenagers) especially tend to start developing bad habits, like not having a regular bedtime. Here are some tips for improving sleep.

- If your child does not wake up spontaneously in the morning, he or she might not be getting enough sleep.
- Different kids have different sleep needs. Look for clues such as fussiness and irritability as signs that your child is not getting enough sleep.
- Take TV or video games or other high-energy activities out of the bedroom. It's best for the bedroom to be a haven, a relaxing place where your child knows he or she can go to wind down.
- Have a regular bedtime. If your child is tired during the daytime, make bedtime 15 or 30 minutes earlier.
- Use a consistent bedtime routine, such as a bath or shower, a story or reading, and a few minutes of cuddling or talking to help your child or teenager wind down. Our bodies respond to outside signals to relax.
- Avoid caffeine, especially in the afternoon or evening.

If you notice that your child is tired during the daytime, especially if you have already tried all of these tips, see your pediatrician. Like overweight adults, overweight children can develop sleep apnea, a condition in which impaired breathing creates a wakeful state. They spend a lot of time in bed but do not get the rest that their bodies and minds need. The doctor will ask if your child snores and has irregular breathing patterns while sleeping.

If these signs are present, or if your child has too much daytime fatigue, your doctor may order a sleep study to evaluate for sleep apnea. It's important to treat sleep apnea if it's present, because good sleep is so critical to the ability to concentrate, complete tasks, be active, and feel good.

Sleep for Teenagers

Teens are often too busy to get enough sleep, but they need it just as much.

- Limit late activities on school nights.
- Set a reasonable "lights out" time. They don't have to sleep, but they don't get to have the TV, video games, cell phone, or lights on.
- Teach the importance of good sleep habits by being a good role model.
- Teenagers need a lot more sleep than they realize—and don't function well early in the morning. If you can, let them have a time to get up that is a little later (like 8 or 9 a.m.). If school starts really early, then the later time is on the weekends. Don't worry—they grow out of it eventually.

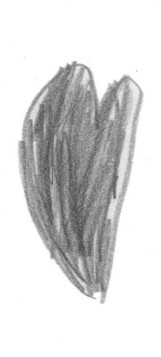

Getting the Very
Sedentary Child Moving

Natalia's mother explained to me that Natalia, just 8 years old, has trouble reaching her feet to put on her shoes. Her mom thinks that her body fat prevents her from bending over. I use a simple test in my clinic: climbing up on the exam table. It's a typical padded table with a step at one end, and when I am ready to do the physical exam, I ask the child to "hop up there." I usually point out the step as well.

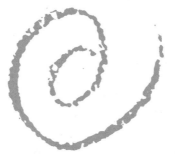

If they are tall enough, some children will stand close to the table and jump up and sit. Many of the overweight children walk to the end of the table, climb up on the step, and then slide over. Some kids have trouble getting to the middle of the table. Some kids can't sit up after they have lain down to be examined. This is a very worrisome sign. Natalia was in this category. To sit up, she had to roll over to her side and push herself up with her hands. She couldn't do even the equivalent of one sit-up. This type of muscle weakness is the beginning of a vicious cycle. She has less muscle to move herself around, so she will move less, have more injuries, and then, she will gain more weight.

If your child does not move and has trouble sitting up like Natalia, seek outside help. I suggest talking to your pediatrician about physical therapy, if it is available, and joining some sort of organized sport. Swimming is a good activity for the very overweight child and so is weight lifting—great places to start. If you decide to have a personal trainer or someone else help you, make sure that they are experienced in working with children and that they use a positive, encouraging, supportive approach.

Starting a new physical activity is a lot like pushing a sled over the snow. The biggest effort is at the beginning—to loosen the sled from the grip of the ice and get it moving. Once it's moving, the sled glides along with little effort. Getting your child and yourself moving will probably be a little like this. The first time you go walking or to a new community/fitness center, it will be unfamiliar and even a little scary. But it gets much easier and more fun over time.

Advice from the Exercise Physiologist

Dr. Steve Reichman works with overweight adults and studies how they benefit from exercise. He has noticed that everyone responds differently. You can't compare your child's activity with that of another child. You have to look at what your child needs. It's pretty simple. If your child is in a phase of too much weight gain, she or he probably needs more activity. If you have a child who does very little, adding one hour a day of playing outside or walking to the park and back will make a big difference.

Dr. Reichman also says that the activity needs to be social. In his research studies on physical activity, his overweight patients show up three or more times a week to exercise. He says they "push them pretty hard," but almost everyone stays and completes the study. How does he do it? Dr. Reichman thinks it's because it's social. His patients meet in groups of five or six and exercise together. They talk while working out and bond with each other. He says if someone is late or not there, the others call and check on them. The friendship part of their exercise program is a big reason that gets them there. So, he recommends that you focus on social and fun activities and not solitary things for your child. Good ideas are playing ball, walking in groups, and dance classes.

Dr. Reichman tells his own kids (ages 8, 6, 4, and 2) that "the TV will suck your brains out." Of course, this isn't true, but too much time in front of the TV will suck the life out of your family. He says that when the TV is off and his kids are in the family room, one is playing ball, the other running in circles, with another trying to get the ball. As soon as the TV goes on, they freeze, sit down, and begin staring forward at the screen. All activity stops.

If you have a child who is naturally sedentary, you will need to be extra careful about TV use. Some families I work with choose to make TV a weekend-only activity. Others limit it to 30 minutes per day. With younger kids, an easy solution is the 30-minute DVD, and then you have no arguing over choosing to watch the next show.

Go Somewhere

I live in a walking community. Many people move here because they want to walk to school, church, and the grocery store. Look at a map of your neighborhood. Are you driving to places that are closer than 1 mile to your house—a store, school, or friend's house? If you have not been walking with your child, having a place to go helps. The next time, put on your walking shoes and walk there together. This is walking for the purpose of going somewhere. That's a strong motivator.

Starting Exercise for the Very Overweight Child

If your child (or you) is very overweight, getting started in physical activity takes some planning, but it will be worth it! If your child wants to go to the gym, Dr. Reichman suggests strength training. You remember that one of the benefits of building more muscles is that muscles burn three times more calories than fat. Weight lifting is something almost every child can do, and overweight children can be better at it than their peers. This is another activity that you might join your child in doing. After some weeks of success with weights, you can add something else, such as brisk walks or bike rides. If you have little experience with these types of activities, find a program or trainer at your local gym or YMCA to help you. There is one basic rule: start out slow and stay with it over the long term. Most benefits will be seen after 6 months or even a year.

Another good activity for a young person who is very overweight is water-based exercise. Playing games in the pool can be fun and is great exercise, too. Many Ys and fitness and community centers have water aerobics.

Finally, walking is available to almost everyone. If your son or daughter (or you) gets out of breath quickly, then begin by walking just one or two blocks the first few times. Increase the walk by a small amount (1–2 blocks) each week. This can be a nice time to talk with your child, observe nature, do some errands, and enjoy the walking.

Sharing the Power:
3 Ps and 3 Cs

Coauthored by Jennifer Buechner, RD, CSP

Keisha and Darryl found family meals to be very stressful. Every dinner seemed like a struggle. They had two children. Two-year-old Deshawn was a picky eater, and his pediatrician pointed out his small size at each well-child check-up. But his 8-year-old sister Nicole had never been small and now she was rapidly gaining weight. Keisha and Darryl spent each dinnertime trying to get Deshawn to eat, while monitoring the amount Nicole was eating. They never enjoyed their own dinners. They loved their kids dearly and were worried about them both. They also felt bad, that as parents, they didn't seem to be meeting everyone's expectations for helping their children to be the right size.

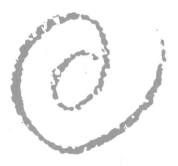

Dinnertime looked like popcorn popping. Deshawn wouldn't stay in his seat. Darryl and Keisha spent half the meal bringing him back to the table. Keisha usually ended up back in the kitchen fixing Deshawn his favorite food, macaroni and cheese, just to get him to eat. Nicole got upset in the process. "It's not fair! I like macaroni and cheese, too, but all I get is this little piece of chicken and all these vegetables!" Keisha knew Nicole had a point but felt that Nicole just needed to get used to eating healthy food. She knew that Nicole was sneaking food because she had found candy wrappers in Nicole's backpack the week before, when she was looking for the PTA newsletter.

Many parents become frustrated with feeding and regard meals as a chore to be handled like cleaning and laundry . . . just get it over with. Sometimes, parents have very different ideas about the roles they play in feeding their children and end up at odds. When I ask parents if they enjoy mealtime with their kids, many of them look at me like I'm crazy.

Consistency at the Table

Like many parents, Keisha and Darryl felt that they had to use different feeding strategies for each child because they were so different. However, it actually works better to use one consistent approach, even if you have five extremely different personalities and body types. Using one approach eliminates jealousy and resentment.

Nicole was jealous that Deshawn was given foods that she wasn't allowed to have. If this continued, she might become resentful of her little brother as well as of her parents' restrictions. Like most 2-year-olds, Deshawn was smart. He knew he could work his parents to get what he wanted. He also had a false sense of power, because he got things his sister didn't. Beware the 2-year-old who learns the art of manipulation; things only get worse! In the short-term, Deshawn went to bed with food in his stomach and Nicole seemed to eat "appropriate" portions of healthy foods. But mom and dad left the table frazzled and unsatisfied with their own meals. In the long run Deshawn will probably become pickier and his table behavior intolerable because he was being "rewarded" for his behavior with macaroni and cheese. Restricting Nicole from eating foods she liked in satisfying portions was already backfiring because she was sneaking food.

Challenges like this are very common, and much of it relates to parenting style. In fact, Keisha and Darryl were using two very different parenting styles for their kids. With Deshawn, they were being "indulgent." In an effort to get him to eat, they catered to his whims. With Keisha, they were restrictive.

We taught Keisha, Darryl, and Nicole how to share control of what Nicole ate at meals using the 3 Ps and the 3 Cs. These letters stand for the roles and responsibilities of the parents and the children when it comes to food and eating. The 3 Ps for parents and 3 Cs for children are based on the work of Ellyn Satter, MS, RD.[29–31] The 3 Ps and 3 Cs are practical, real actions that each of you can do to improve mealtimes in your family.

Keisha and Darryl were skeptical about giving their kids control of how much they ate. They were having a hard time getting one child to eat enough and the other not to eat too much. And here I was, asking them to allow their kids to choose how much they ate or whether they ate at all.

Keisha and Darryl had to learn to trust that their kids' inborn ability to eat wisely would take over when everyone settled into the new pattern. When they started using the 3 Ps and 3 Cs, Deshawn threw fits when he didn't get what he wanted. Nicole ate larger portions in the beginning, in response to her new freedom to choose how much to eat. The parents were nervous, but hung in there, doing their own jobs without trying to take over their kids' jobs.

Within a few weeks, the atmosphere at the family dinner table had changed. There were no more fights. Meals were served family style and at scheduled times. Deshawn seemed proud that he was learning to serve himself, and he ate more

The 3 Ps and 3 Cs

3 Ps for Parents:

Plan for positives
Prepare and put food on the table
Provide with patience

3 Cs for Children:

From the dishes parents put on the table, **the children:**
Choose what they will eat
Choose how much they will eat
Choose if they will eat

Planning for positives includes:
- planning what to shop for
- planning what will be served at meals and snacks
- deciding where food can be eaten in the house
- planning what times meals and snacks will be served

Preparing and putting food on the table includes:
- deciding which foods go on the table
- presenting meals and snacks on the table
- determining what menu items can be ordered when eating out

Providing with patience includes:
- sitting and eating with your kids
- supporting them in their efforts to learn new skills and manners . . . without pressure
- role modeling how you would like them to eat and act at the table
- allowing your toddler to make a mess while she learns how to get food into her mouth, with or without utensils
- keeping mealtimes pleasant

©Stress Free Feeding Program, Children's Healthcare of Atlanta.

of what he chose to put on his plate. Nicole chatted pleasantly instead of pouting, and her pace of eating slowed down. The kids weren't eating perfectly, but they weren't eating any worse, and there was no more conflict at the table. They were on their way. A few months later, Deshawn was starting to try some new foods on his own, and Nicole was no longer sneaking food.

Forbidden Foods

Keely's grandfather died from a heart attack when she was very young. Her parents were interested in avoiding this genetic tendency for heart disease and to ensure good health for themselves and for Keely. Around the time Keely was 6 years old, her parents decided to put the family on a very-low-fat diet. They drank fat-free milk and ate only lean meat. They carefully restricted the portions of food that went onto Keely's plate at dinner times so she wouldn't be able to overeat. Foods that were high in fat were forbidden in the house. She wasn't allowed to buy school lunches; she could only eat what was in her lunch box. For the most part, Keely did okay. But at her friends' houses, she would eat things she knew she shouldn't have. When her parents weren't home, she would eat as much as she could—bingeing on forbidden foods.

Keely is a young lady now, and she represents a different end of the spectrum of weight-related food problems. In their enthusiasm to reduce fat and portion sizes for improving health, her parents inadvertently hurt Keely in some ways. The restrictive approach ended up being unhealthy. She internalized their fear of food and became overly concerned with "eating healthy." This helped to set her up for a later struggle with an eating disorder. She became a skillful dieter, beginning in high school. She learned the calorie content of every food. By her sophomore year of college, Keely had tried a liquid protein diet, a no-carbohydrate diet, a high-fiber low-carbohydrate diet, the ice cream diet, the 5-foods diet, the 500-calorie diet, the 1000-calorie diet, the grapefruit diet, and an egg-chicken-prunes diet.

It's not surprising that Keely developed problems with food. Medical research shows that strictly controlling food and banning foods can lead to overeating later and sometimes even eating disorders. The role of parents in feeding their children is deeply tied to nurturing and loving the child. Even though Keely's mom and dad restricted certain foods because they thought it was the best thing, it felt like punishment to Keely, because she left the table hungry and deprived of the simple satisfaction that comes from eating. Sneaking food because she was hungry made her feel worse. Parents and children each have important roles in feeding and eating. But Keely didn't get to carry out her responsibility, which is to eat the amount of food she needed at the dinner table.

3 Cs: Children Can Choose

Children are born with the ability to listen and respond to the messages their bodies give them about hunger and fullness. Normal infants have an excellent internal sense of how many calories they need. They can naturally regulate how much to eat. As I explained in the chapter on growth (Chapter 2), your baby will eat more during growth spurts and then, at other times, is content to sleep more and eat less often. They know when they are hungry and when they are full.

Being disconnected from this "knowing" can begin very early, such as when someone urges a baby to take more formula than the baby wants. It may happen later when a parent of an overweight child restricts how much she or he eats at a meal.

Are you able to eat when you are hungry and stop when you are full? Or do you feel out of control with your eating? Many people are somewhere in between. When we pay more attention to the external "shoulds" and "should nots" of eating, we are separated from our inborn ability to regulate ourselves. The wonderful thing is that kids and adults who have lost this internal sense can get it back. It's easier to do when a child is younger, but it's possible to restore internal regulation even in adults who have become extremely disconnected from their body through years of weight control efforts.

When kids are restricted from eating, they start to worry that they won't get enough. When specific restricted foods are available, children will often overeat them. One study showed that preschool girls who are restricted at home eat more than twice the amount of "tasty" foods (high in fat and sugar) than unrestricted girls do when given a chance.[32]

When some kids are pressured to eat, they eat less. It doesn't matter if it's positive pressure (This spinach will make you strong!) or negative pressure. (If you don't finish your food, you won't be able to go out to play.) Pressuring a child to eat backfires, just as restricting foods backfires because both interfere with the child's ability to self-regulate. When kids lose the connection to their own appetite as the primary motivation to eat or not eat, their weight becomes unstable.

In fact, breastfeeding supports an infant's ability to self-regulate. Breastfeeding is an example of a child feeding without pressure. You can't measure how much the baby takes; the baby decides. Probably in part because of this, breast-feeding exclusively for the first 2 months of life reduces the likelihood of your child becoming overweight during child-hood. If you can breastfeed until the baby is 6 months of age, you increase the chances that your baby will be obesity-free until adolescence.[33]

It's not a good idea to focus on getting your children to clean their plates. "Cleaning your plate" was the rule when food was a lot of work to produce and was precious. Now food is plentiful, even excessive in many households. The bigger danger now is not that your child won't get enough food, but that she or he will eat too much.

Tips on Supporting Self-Regulation

- Trust your baby when she stops feeding or slows down. If she seems hungry, even though it's "not time yet," she might just be hungry. Let her decide.
- If you bottle feed, watch for cues that your baby is finished with a feeding. Don't encourage finishing the bottle just to keep from wasting formula. Babies may take different amounts at different feedings; this is normal.

⟲ Likewise, trust your child to know to stop eating when he is done and don't pressure him to finish up. To avoid wasting food, ask your child to start with small servings; he or she can always have more.

⟲ Don't bring snacks with you everywhere. Errands and excursions that take 2 or 3 hours are good times to go without eating. Don't stop to buy food if you will be home soon to eat a planned snack or dinner.

⟲ Your child can rediscover the ability to self-regulate—to know when she is hungry and when she is full. Focus on enhancing this inborn ability through supportive mealtime experiences and a consistent family meal and snack structure.

Foods that Can Hurt Self-Regulation

Can we blame high-sugar, high-fat foods for the increase in childhood obesity? Foods that are highly desirable—because they are very sweet or have lots of fat—can overwhelm a child's internal sense of being full (satisfied). This is especially true if they are served frequently or completely restricted. Most studies suggest that children have pretty accurate self-regulating systems: they decrease the amount of calories they eat later if they eat a lot earlier. Your activities can influence this. For example, restricting foods make them more desirable. And we know that we seek and eat more of the things that are desirable. However, serving them all the time doesn't work either.

So, what's the best way to handle tasty high-sugar, high-fat foods? Only buy and serve them occasionally. (This is the same reason to eat out only occasionally.) If these foods are not in your house, then it is easier to not eat them every day. Also, many of these foods are relatively expensive—another good reason to not buy them.

To avoid making packaged foods too precious in your children's minds, let them eat all they want when you do serve

them. Don't worry—it balances
out over the week and will help
them not to binge in the future.
For example, if you have been
completely limiting soda, serve
it with lunch on Saturday. Buy
one two-liter bottle and let everyone have as much as they want
until the bottle is empty. The first
time your children will probably

Examples of Packaged Foods Marketed to Kids

- Potato chips
- Cake and cookie snacks
- Sodas
- Sweetened cereal
- Juice-like beverages

drink a lot. Plan it again the next Saturday—and again let
them have as much as they want. After a while it will become
routine and less special, and they may even decrease the
amount that they take. If there is a food that your child begs
for, you will decrease its value by providing it on a regular
schedule.

Setting Limits

Kids need and expect limits. Setting limits is part of good
parenting, but it's harder to do than it seems. It is a balancing act, and it's best to avoid extremes. Parents who set clear,
reasonable limits and consistently and kindly follow through
with negative consequences when children exceed those limits,
create a healthy environment. Making strict rules that are
unreasonable or having very few rules, or rules that can be
bent or argued out of, will backfire. When kids are pushing
your buttons, you will want to give in, but you will end up
losing a great deal. As the parent, you have to decide on the
rules you want everyone to live by and then stick to them.
If dinner is planned for 5:30 and your child is whining at
5:15 because she's hungry, explain to her that she can wait
a little longer.

It's okay to be hungry. Help your child learn to identify
this feeling. You could say, "I know you are hungry. Dinner
will be ready at 5:30. That's just 15 more minutes. Would you
like to color a picture for me while you are waiting?" Identify

the feeling, reinforce that food is predictable and on schedule, and help your child develop a strategy to cope with the feeling.

In general, both extremes of parenting—too permissive and too restrictive—can lead to weight problems in children. There is a fine line, and the biggest challenge of parenting is to stay in that middle ground of appropriate limits and structure while allowing your child to explore, develop, and grow.

I was talking to one of my graduate students about food restriction and the long-term harm it can have. She seemed a little uncomfortable. "At the dinner table, sometimes we divide up one of the items for our kids," she said, and then explained, "If we have something special, it needs to go all the way around the table." She and her husband have four young children, all under the age of 8 years old, and when they sit down to dinner, the parents make sure that each child gets a chance for each item, otherwise the first two might take all of something. I quickly reassured her that this behavior is part of learning to eat politely with your family. That's not restrictive. It's appropriate limit setting.

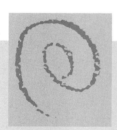

Question for the Psychologist

Q **My husband really wants our kids to eat all the food on their plates. But I want them to eat just the amount they want and then not let them have anything else until snack time like Dr. Vos said. How do I get him to "buy in"?**

A Have you talked it over with him? Find out why he wants the plates clean. See if you and he can come up with a plan that satisfies both of you. Studies show that if kids serve themselves, they take smaller portions. Is he willing to let the kids serve themselves, with some simple guidelines, such as, "Start with a little. You can get more if you are still hungry."

The Problem with Diets

Adults who lose weight as part of a very-low-calorie diet, on average, regain 115% of their weight within 5 years.[34] In other words, they weigh more than they did before they started the diet! Doctors seem to be going about obesity treatment all wrong, telling patients and families to give up what they really like—the food they like, the activities they like. Overweight patients are encouraged to *sacrifice* in order to improve their short- or long-term health.[35] Many weight-loss therapies ask patients to severely restrict themselves. However, food restriction by parents leads to sneaking and bingeing in children. Does self-restriction lead to the same things? Many people do develop this pattern. They are very "good" for a while, and then they binge on the thing that they have been wanting. Next, they feel bad about that, and soon they have "given up."

There are several ways you can avoid this cycle for your child. First, use healthier lifestyle habits and not a short-term diet. Most children will stabilize and even improve their health and weight by watching less TV, drinking less sugary drinks, playing outside more, and being served wholesome foods. You can teach your child to be proud and happy in the body he or she has so that your child doesn't start restricting and bingeing.

It is true that most adults who lose weight will regain it over the long term.[36] The good news for you is that young children and children in general have the best chance of maintaining improvements in weight. Why is this? I think it's for several reasons. First, children are still growing. Getting healthier is often a matter of keeping weight steady while height naturally increases (see Chapter 3). And, children are more flexible metabolically compared with adults (see Chapter 4). But most important, kids have your support—the support of their moms, dads, grandfathers, grandmothers, aunts, uncles, cousins, brothers, and sisters. By making healthy changes as a family, you can support, motivate, and problem-solve together for long-term success.

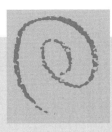

Question for the Psychologist

Q **I thought I heard my teenage daughter vomiting. I am worried that she might have an eating disorder. She is really thin. Should I talk to her, and what should I watch out for?**

A It is common for young people to develop unhealthy food habits in response to peer and culture pressures and as a way of coping with emotional difficulties. What they do not realize is that these habits can be addictive, trapping them in a sickness they cannot overcome without help. One type of eating disorder consists of restricting food intake, sometimes to the point of starvation (anorexia). Another type consists of bingeing on great quantities of food and then getting rid of it by vomiting or using laxatives (bulimia). These two types can also be combined, where the person is underweight and practices bingeing and purging.

It would be good for you to express your concern to your daughter in a gentle way. Ask if she is worried about her weight and what she knows about eating disorders. If your daughter does not think of herself as fat when she really is thin (anorexia), she may not have an eating disorder. However, because she is so thin, I would recommend that she have an appointment for a physical check-up. If she is underweight, her doctor will see if there is an underlying physical problem, suggest ways to gain some weight, and, if necessary, refer her to a counselor trained in eating disorders. If she thinks she is fat, she has a belief that is typical of people with anorexia. Speak with her doctor about this, who will decide if a referral to a psychologist is needed.

Children with bulimic problems can be hard to spot, because they usually are not underweight and tend to be clever about hiding the bingeing and purging. If your daughter has a habit of going directly to the bathroom after eating or if she eats great quantities of food and is not overweight, I suggest you ask some friendly questions about these habits. If she denies purging, and you still suspect something, just keep observing. If there is a problem, you will find evidence sooner or later. In that case, it is also important to take your daughter to a counselor trained in eating disorders. Expect to be asked to take part in family therapy, as this is an important part of the treatment of eating disorders.

Ps and Cs: The Bottom Line

It is your role as the parent *to create a structure of meals and snacks and to offer healthy foods.* Your child's role is *to choose what to eat within that structure.* You need to trust that you can do this and have fun with it. Your child does not need a "perfect" diet in order to have the healthiest body. Remember:

- Don't short-order cook or make substitutes during dinner.
- Ignore all the ads that say picky eaters are normal and that you need to buy special products they say your child will love.
- Plan meals around food that you enjoy, not just what you think you "ought to eat."
- Accept your child's size and shape, and you won't have a hidden agenda.
- Find a positive reason to make changes, such as to enjoy your meals and each other's company.

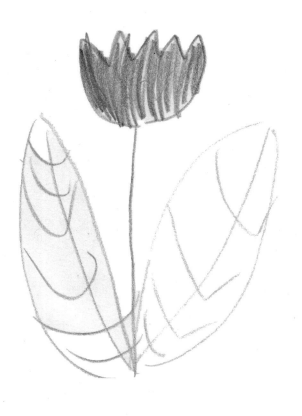

12

Drinking Water and Reducing Sugar

I asked my cousin R, who teaches classes for personal trainers and coaches and has three young kids of her own, "What would it take for you to stop giving your children soda? What would motivate you?" I asked because she had just reassured me that they only gave their kids caffeine-free sodas, and I thought that was interesting. It's common to focus on the potential harmfulness of the caffeine in sodas—but not the sugar. In fact, R and her husband give their kids only one soda a week, but she herself has a daily soda as an afternoon treat. She realized that soon, as the kids got older, it may be hard to limit them to one soda without addressing the number of sodas that she and her husband drink.

R said she does worry about the kids' constant exposure to sugar. "But to fix it, you have to change the culture," she said, "It's everywhere." She described the snacks at a recent hockey game for her 7-year-old. The kids were given Gatorade and a bag of candy after the game. "What do you do at that point?" asked her husband. "Take it away? Make a spectacle when all the other kids are chowing down?" They were concerned about sugary drinks and snacks being routine at children's sport events, and I agree. Young children don't need sports drinks, which can have as much sugar as a soda. One of the authors of the book *The Fattening of America* (see Resources) coaches his son's soccer team, and calls himself a "tyrant coach" because he only allows water and fruit at games. This is excellent. Maybe he and other concerned parents like my cousin will start a new culture where water and fruit are the norm. I just ran a 5 K race, and at the finish, they handed out chunks of banana and bottles of water instead of the usual sports drinks. That's perfect!

It has been proven that the more sugar you eat, the more sugar you need in order to taste it. Adapting to the amount of sugar in a food happens in the few minutes it takes to eat a bowl of sweetened yogurt; the first bite tastes much sweeter than the last.[37] This also occurs over a longer time. Perhaps you used to use two packets of sweetener in your coffee, but now it takes four or five for it to taste the way you like.

Americans consume much higher levels of sugar and sweeteners than ever before. We drink 55 gallons of soda per person each year. This one behavior plays a leading role in why our children get too many calories.

Reclaiming Your Family's Sense of Taste

One problem with eating so many sugary foods is that it screws up your sense of taste. The best way to regain a real sensitivity to sweet flavors is to stop eating sweetened foods for a while. Then smaller amounts of sugar will satisfy your taste, and you will be able to enjoy the natural sweetness in

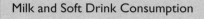

Milk and Soft Drink Consumption

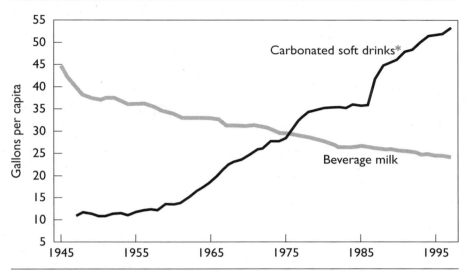

*1947 is the first year for which data on soft drink consumption are available.
Source: USDA/Economic Research Service. From www.ers.usda.gov. Accessed January 25, 2008.

many foods. A sun-ripened tomato, a fresh ear of corn on the cob, and even Bibb lettuce all have sweetness. Milk is actually quite high in a natural sugar—lactose—which has a sweet taste. In fact, you can use powdered milk as a substitute for some of the sugar in recipes. Milk also has protein and other nutrients that white sugar lacks. Over time, I have decreased my own consumption of sweetened foods. I used to put some sugar in my coffee or drink a chai latte (with honey in it). Now, I am quite sensitive to the sweetness of milk because it is often the only sweet thing I have early in the day. I drink a latte coffee (espresso with steamed milk), and it tastes sweet to me because of the milk.

Large amounts of sugar may interfere with the taste of other flavors as well. A TV-show host told me what his teenage daughter had discovered about this. His daughter had given up soft drinks for Lent and—to her surprise—found that she could taste all of her food better. I think that this is a great reason not to drink soft drinks with meals. They make it harder to taste and enjoy your other food and could decrease your ability to judge how much to eat.

Sodas and Sweetened Beverages

One of the best changes that my patients make is to limit soda and sugar-sweetened beverages—and to drink water instead. Most children in my clinic tell me that they drink three to four sodas or sweetened beverages *every day*. This is 24 to 32 ounces of sugary drinks or 800 to 1000 calories per day—*half of what that child needs to eat for the day.* No wonder parents tell me that it doesn't really seem like their children eat that much. They are drinking half or more of their calories.

There are several problems with sugar calories in drinks. One is that the body doesn't seem to recognize them as nourishment. Sugar from a drink is rapidly absorbed, so it doesn't satisfy for long. The sugar from drinks increases cavities in your child's teeth. It can slow your child's growth because most of these beverages are not a source of calcium. In fact, the more sugar-sweetened beverages a child drinks, the more likely he or she is to be deficient in calcium, which is necessary for growing taller and stronger bones.

Simple Changes to Reduce Sugar

- Limit soda and sugar-sweetened beverages to planned occasions (in my house, we had soda when we had pizza, usually on Friday nights).
- It's easier if sodas aren't in the house, so don't buy them regularly.
- Your kids will want to drink what they see you drinking. Be a role model.
- Try having fun cups and straws when you switch to water.
- When you do have them, water down sugary beverages, so your children get used to drinking things that are "less sweet."

◎ Teens and some younger children might enjoy a slice of lemon or lime in ice water as a refreshing summer drink.

◎ If they are truly thirsty, they will drink what's offered. Don't worry if they walk away when offered water. They'll be back when they *are* thirsty.

Artificial Sweeteners

Diet sodas and many other foods contain artificial sweeteners. Families making changes, like decreasing sugar, often ask me what I think about artificial sweeteners. One of my issues with them is that they haven't been studied well enough in young

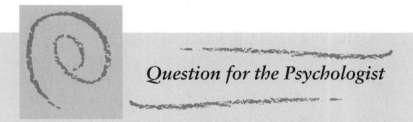

Question for the Psychologist

Q **What if I want to stop buying sodas but my husband refuses to do without them? He drinks three or four a day, and he is at least 40 pounds overweight so the change would benefit him, too.**

A It is hard when a parenting partner resists our efforts to make healthy changes. You can only accept his decision and make the best of it. Much as we may want to make somebody else conform to what we think is best, and however right we may be, we cannot make somebody else do something. Your husband likes to drink sodas and does not want anyone telling him to stop. If you have not done so already, ask him nicely if he will please consider stopping for the sake of the kids. If his answer is no, or his behavior says no, then you'll need to work around this problem. You could ask him not to drink sodas in front of the kids, because they are not allowed to drink as many as he does. You could teach the kids that, because dad is dad, he gets to decide for himself if he wants to follow the doctor's advice. They, however, are kids, and they have to go by what mom says, at least until they are adults, too. Kids will accept this.

children. There are no 10- and 20-year studies of the effects of artificial sweeteners in children. A child's growing body is not like an adult's. You wouldn't give children large amounts of caffeine or alcohol. I think artificial sweeteners are in the same category. They are not nutritionally necessary or beneficial. My bottom-line advice is to avoid artificial sweeteners in your child's food.

There is some evidence that artificial sweeteners may not be that healthy. Animal studies of appetite have shown that artificial sweeteners interrupt a rat's ability to sense how many calories it is eating.[38] Like most animals, rats are normally very good at eating just what they need to stay at a healthy weight. But in these studies, scientists found that they could easily confuse the rats by switching from sweet-tasting sugary foods to sweet-tasting artificially sweetened foods. After this, the rats lost the ability to eat only what they needed and ate too much regular food, eventually becoming obese.

The Framingham Study followed a large group of normal, healthy adults over time. In one part of the study, researchers collected information about diet and then measured risk factors for cardiovascular disease 4 years later. They found that those who reported drinking one soda a day had twice the risk of developing obesity, high blood pressure, and high cholesterol, compared with those who had a soda only occasionally. The most striking finding was that *the diet soda drinkers had the exact same risks of obesity as the regular soda drinkers*.[39] At first, this doesn't make sense, because the diet drinkers don't take in all those extra calories. Although this study did not show why diet sodas didn't "work," the researchers proposed that the sweetness of the diet drinks may create a taste preference for highly sweetened foods. Therefore, diet soda drinkers may be seeking out sweeter foods.

Frequent soda drinking also seems to be a signal for a group of unhealthy habits. In other words, someone who drinks soda is more likely to eat less fiber[40] and drink less milk and to be less active.[41] In the Framingham Study, those who drank soda were more likely to smoke as well. This doesn't mean that an occasional diet drink will hurt your child, but I would recommend not making it a daily habit.

The Benefits of Water

Water is the most thirst-quenching beverage you can give your child.[42] If you drink a water-sugar mixture, only about 60% of the water is available for the body. But if you drink water, 100% of it is available.

- Water is the most thirst-quenching beverage.
- Water is the least expensive beverage (tap water).
- Water is available almost everywhere.
- Water doesn't cause health problems (in normal amounts).
- Water flushes out the body and the kidneys.

Water is necessary to every living creature. It regulates body temperature; moistens tissues, such as those in the mouth, eyes, and nose; lubricates joints; protects body organs and tissues; helps prevent constipation; lessens the burden on the kidneys and liver by flushing out waste products; and helps dissolve nutrients and minerals so the body can use them.

How much do you need to drink each day? The answer is not as simple as you might think. Your water needs depend on many factors, including your health, how active you are, and where you live. Your child is probably drinking enough water if he or she doesn't complain of feeling thirsty and his or her urine is colorless or slightly yellow.

Adults who supervise children and teens in physical activities should make sure they drink water before, during, and after exercise. Water is the best fluid for children and doesn't need to be very cold. It's easier to drink if it's not full of ice.

Water is found in a variety of foods and beverages. Our food provides about 20% of our total daily amount of water. The remaining 80% comes from drinking water and other beverages. Foods that are extra high in water are watermelons and cucumbers, which are nearly 100% water by weight. Beverages such as milk and juice are also mostly water.

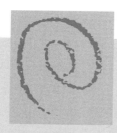

Question for the Psychologist

Q **My sister and her daughter are both really overweight, and they drink lots of soda at home. Can I say something to her?**

A If you have a good relationship with your sister, say something in a respectful way. Use an "I feel" statement to tell her about your concern: "I worry about how you and your daughter drink lots of sodas, because I learned that sodas put more extra pounds on people than almost any other food or drink." Your sister may not have realized this connection and be willing to try cutting down on the sodas. Or she may not want to hear it. It is her choice to make.

What About Juice?

On a recent trip to Mexico, I ate breakfast at the hotel restaurant buffet. It was an amazing spread with lots of familiar and unfamiliar foods. In the beverage area, there was a large metal press with a bowl of orange halves to the left of it. I decided to try it, got a glass and half an orange, and set to work. I put the orange half between the lever and the round knob and began to squeeze it together, but it was really hard and not much juice came out. Luckily, the server saw what I was doing and ran over, removed my orange and turned it upside down— the juice ran into my glass easily. The glass I had was a typical 16-ounce water glass. When I squeezed two halves of one orange, I ended up with just a few ounces of juice in the bottom. It was delicious.

Nearby was a dispenser of juices. While I was busy squeezing one orange, several people had filled their glasses at the machine with 16 ounces of thick, processed orange juice. A typical 16-ounce glass of orange juice contains the juice of 3 to 4 oranges and 11 teaspoons of natural sugar. My medium-sized orange resulted in just a few ounces of juice with 3 to 4 teaspoons of sugar, along with 4 grams of fiber to help fill me up.

Juice is fine in small amounts. Most pediatricians recommend that children be introduced to juice in the second half of the first year but only an ounce or two a day.[43] If you are trying to reduce the amount of sugar your family eats, consider not buying juice regularly. Even 100% juice has three to four times the amount of sugar than is in a piece of fruit. It can be healthy in small amounts along with plenty of water and milk.

Instead of offering juice, you can offer a piece of fruit and a glass of water. Whole fruit has more fiber and is more filling than juice. Wash the fruit to remove any chemicals from the growing process. The peel is a healthy source of fiber, so it's better to teach your family to eat fruit with the peel in the case of apples, peaches, and pears. Remove the peel for toddlers until they have enough ability to chew it.

Tip for Serving Juice

To serve juice, try to find some old-fashioned little juice glasses. Remember those little 3- and 4-ounce plastic juice glasses we all used to have? It can be challenging to find them (see Resources), but it really helps to have the right size glass just for juice. If juice goes in a big glass, your child will likely pour and drink too much.

Juice Guidelines

- No juice before 6 months of age.
- Do not give infants juice in bottles or travel cups. They should not drink juice throughout the day.
- Do not give infants juice at bedtime.
- For children aged 1 to 6 years, limit juice to 4 to 6 ounces per day.
- For children aged 7 to 18 years, limit juice to 8 to 12 ounces per day.
- Encourage children to eat whole fruits.

Source: Reference 43.

Sports Drinks

Sports drinks work by increasing water transfer from the stomach into the bloodstream, where it is needed, through the exchange of salt and glucose. Fructose and glucose (sugars) are added to sports drinks because they are rapid sources of energy. Fructose does not stimulate an insulin peak that could cause fatigue an hour later. Sports drinks were designed for professional adult athletes engaged in extremely physical and prolonged activity. There is no reason to use them in short moderate- or low-level activity, especially in children.

- Sports rehydration drinks are recommended for events lasting *over 2 hours* or *in extreme heat.*
- True rehydration drinks should not taste sweet.
- If you buy a full-sugar sports drink, add water to make it more hydrating.
- Buy the powdered version of the drink and mix it in your own bottle using one third more water than called for.
- Offer your child water and a piece of fruit after exercise. You can't beat that for convenience and health.
- Don't offer sports drinks at non-sports occasions.

How Can Parents Change the Culture?

Going back to the soda question, I think my cousin R was right on. It isn't fair for parents to regularly drink soda and then tell the kids they can't have it. There has to be a balance, and each family must find its own approach. Having sodas as an occasional treat is one way. Making sodas forbidden will only increase the attraction and can lead to your child bingeing when he or she gets the chance.

- Talk with other parents about sugar and your concerns.
- If it's your turn to provide the snacks, bring fruit and water.
- Ask your child's teacher not to use candy as a reward for the classroom; options are stickers, homework "passes," bouncy balls, or fancy pencils.

◎ Eat and drink what you want your child to eat and drink.

◎ Have sugary beverages occasionally so that they are not "forbidden." Let your child have as much as he or she wants at that time (or their fair share if the supply is limited).

"Everyone needs a brownie now and then." One of my colleagues said this to me, and I completely agree. Often in my clinic, a parent will tell me that they are definitely going to stop buying ice cream, candy, or some other specific treat. When I researched sources of sugar in the diet of children, dairy products such as ice cream provided only 7% of the fructose and candy provided only 10%. Most of the sugar comes from other foods. In fact, the two biggest categories containing sugar were drinks and processed foods like cereal, cakes, pies, and bread.

Breakfast Cereals

Because I research sugar, I am a little compulsive about reading labels and avoiding sugar and sweeteners for myself. The last time I sat down to breakfast at my grandmother's table, she offered me some juice, and I said "No, thank you." She offered me a popular presweetened cereal, and I again turned it down. If she hadn't offered some eggs and plain oatmeal, of course I would have had to politely eat the sweet cereal. Because I have stopped eating so much sugar, I am much more sensitive to it. Especially in the morning, I prefer unsweetened foods.

In general, the nutritional quality of breakfast cereals for children is poor. A recent study showed that 66% of cereals for children failed to meet national standards for nutrition, mostly because of too much sugar.[44] That's bad, because cereal is a quick way to eat breakfast, and many children eat these cereals. What can you do? Choose better cereals to bring home. "Better" cereals have more fiber and less sugar and are made with whole grains. The good news is that more of these are available today.

- Read the ingredient label for grams of sugar (see page 172).
- Compare grams of sugar to grams of fiber—I like those with as much fiber as sugar.
- Some high-fiber, low-sugar cereals are
  - Kashi cereals
  - Cheerios (the original version)
  - Bran flakes
  - Plain oatmeal
  - Cream of wheat
- Look for cereals with at least 3 grams of fiber per serving and less than 10 grams of sugar in a serving.

Fructose

Fructose is a very common sugar in processed foods and is also found naturally in fruits, vegetables, and fruit juice. Fructose is added to many processed foods because it makes the food taste sweeter, and high-fructose corn syrup (a source of fructose) improves the quality of processed foods, making them softer and last longer on the shelf. Both high-fructose corn syrup and cane sugar have about 50% of the sugar from fructose (the rest is from glucose) so there isn't much difference between the two in my mind. The real question is, *how much of either type of sugar is safe* for your child?

In the 1960s, scientists studied the metabolism of fructose in animals. Even then, it was clear that fructose had a unique ability to stimulate fat production in the body. Unfortunately, throughout the next several decades, there weren't that many studies on fructose in humans. For a while, diabetes researchers thought fructose might be helpful because it doesn't raise blood glucose levels after you eat it, but subsequent research has shown that fructose can worsen insulin resistance and so shouldn't be used by people with diabetes. Several short studies in adults have shown that fructose can increase the blood levels of triglycerides, so the most recent research is focused on understanding if continued

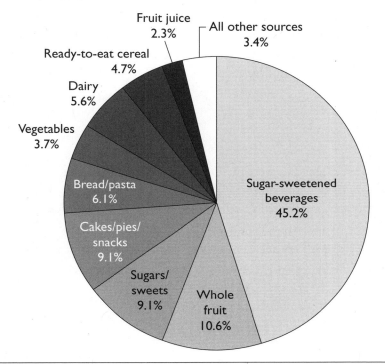

Sources of Fructose for Teens 12 to 18 Years Old

Fruit juice 2.3%

All other sources 3.4%

Ready-to-eat cereal 4.7%

Dairy 5.6%

Vegetables 3.7%

Bread/pasta 6.1%

Cakes/pies/snacks 9.1%

Sugars/sweets 9.1%

Whole fruit 10.6%

Sugar-sweetened beverages 45.2%

Source: Adapted from Vos et al.: Dietary fructose consumption among U.S. children and adults: the Third National Health and Nutrition Examination Survey. *Medscape J Med* 10(7): 160, 2008.

intake is harmful. In children, fructose may be tolerated better because they are active and can adapt to fructose, but there haven't been any good long-term studies of the effects of a diet high in fructose despite its large presence in our food supply.

This pie chart shows that the biggest source of fructose for teenagers is sugary beverages such as soda, juice drinks, and sports drinks. Altogether, the natural sources (fruits, vegetables, and fruit juice) only provide 16.6%. This means that on a typical day, most teenagers would get about 80% less fructose if they didn't consume sugar-sweetened beverages and processed food.

Dessert? Sure, in Moderation

The question of sweets really comes down to moderation. One of the pleasures in life is sweet foods, and everyone should be able to enjoy a dessert or sweet treat on a regular basis. By definition, desserts are usually served after other satisfying foods that are not sweet, so it's harder to eat big portions.

Tips

- Serve dessert in small bowls instead of larger cereal or soup bowls.
- Cut and offer small pieces of dessert for everyone and then offer seconds.
- Make your own lower-sugar, whole-grain desserts.
- Serve fruit for dessert, with some whipped cream or ice cream.
- Make brownies every once in a while, and let everyone enjoy every bite guilt free until they are gone.

I keep a container of dark chocolate discs in the cupboard. I must inherit that gene from my mom because she always has a stash of really good chocolate in a cupboard in her kitchen. In the evening or sometimes for afternoon tea, she will make herbal tea and enjoy a small square of chocolate. It's dark chocolate so it's not as sweet as some kinds and the flavor is rich and strong. Following her tradition, I often have a couple of pieces as my dessert . . . no prep time and immensely enjoyable.

I tell my patients it's okay to have some sugar, it's just not supposed to be in every food item. Sugar belongs in a cookie or cake. It doesn't belong in the spaghetti sauce, the hamburger bun, or the salad dressing. Banning all sweet treats will only make them more desirable for your children and encourage sneaking or bingeing. Better to learn as a family to enjoy sweets in moderation.

Suggestions

- If your family loves a particular dessert, enjoy it once or twice a month—no guilt involved.
- Move most sweet treats to dessert status rather than as part of dinner or snacks. The exception may be whole wheat oatmeal cookies, which I think make a great after-school snack, especially with a glass of milk.
- Make your own cookies and cakes and reduce the sugar in the recipe. You can freeze cookies so they last longer and are available when you need them.
- Kids will be more sensitive to the sweet flavors if the rest of their food isn't sweet.
- Don't serve sweet (diet or regular) beverages with dinner, so everyone can taste their food better and dessert will taste even sweeter.

Sugar, Sugar Everywhere

Sugar can hide on the ingredient label of processed foods because it travels under many names. Here are some names for "sugar" you'll find on the ingredients list of packaged foods. Ask your kids to help you become a label reader and find the culprits! (See a sample food label and get information on how to read it in Chapter 17.)

- Cane sugar
- Dextrose
- Glucose
- Sucrose
- Raw sugar
- Cane syrup
- High-fructose corn syrup
- Corn syrup
- Sugar
- Maltose
- Lactose
- Fruit concentrate

More important than whether there is sugar or not is how much sugar is in the food *per serving*. To help you figure out if there's a lot or a little sugar in a food, convert the "grams of sugar" on the food label to teaspoons. Four grams of sugar equals one teaspoon. If you read the Nutrition Facts on the box of a typical breakfast toaster pastry, you'll see that one pastry has 20 grams of sugar—5 teaspoons! Measure 5 teaspoons of sugar into a dish; you might be surprised.

I don't have fixed standards on how much or how little sugar "should be" in a food. I compare products, and accept more sugar in foods that I think should be sweet. For example, I don't really look at grams of sugar when choosing ice cream. But I do look at grams of sugar when choosing a cereal, crackers, and spaghetti sauce—all foods I prefer not to be sweet.

Check Your Sugar IQ

1. The average jar of spaghetti sauce has _____ grams of sugar per serving.
    a. 0   b. 3   c. 6   d. 12

2. A teaspoon of sugar is the same as _____ grams.

3. True or false? An apple and a glass of apple juice have about the same amount of sugar in them.

4. A typical can of soda has _____ teaspoons of sugar.

5. True or false? Before 1900, sugar was a common source of calories for children and adults.

Answers: 1. c; 2. 4 grams of sugar per teaspoon; 3. False. A 10-ounce glass of juice has three times as much sugar as one apple. 4. 10 teaspoons of sugar per can of soda; 5. False. Sugar became widely available only in the last century.

Reducing sugar in your family's life is a good goal. Combined with more physical activity, doing this can literally save your lives.

Tips for Reducing Sugar

- Make sugary drinks a "sometime" thing, not an everyday item.
- Only have sports drinks after several hours of strenuous physical exertion.
- Provide juice in tiny amounts and not on a daily basis. Reduce the sugar content by adding water.
- Read labels (see Chapter 17). Get your kids to read the labels; they can be your "sugar" sleuths.
- Find cereal and bread with 0 to 2 grams of sugar per serving.
- Buy plain yogurt and add your own jam or fruit to sweeten it.
- If the processed version of the food has sugar in it, make your own without sugar. Look for some great examples in the recipe section.
- Don't go crazy about limiting sugar. Some things should have sugar in them: ice cream, cookies, cakes, candy, and so forth.
- Sodas can be a special occasion item. Use small to medium cups and don't make a big deal out of it. If your children are old enough, let them pour their own.
- Be a good role model, and drink water most of the time.

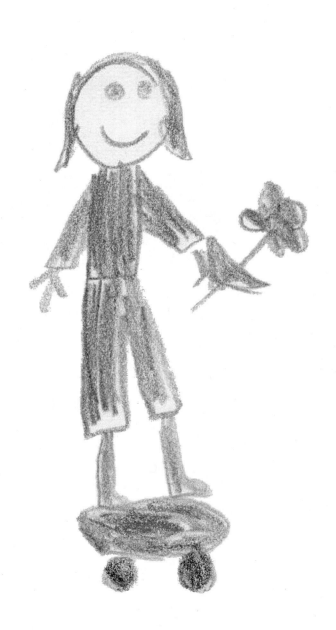

13

Eating Home-Cooked Family Meals

What you feed your children is important. But *how* you feed them may be even more important. Many parents expect me to tell them that their child's health has suffered because they have been allowing the child to eat too much ice cream. I don't know why it's always "ice cream." Actually, ice cream provides calcium and protein—and is very satisfying. The key is to know *when* and *how* to serve the ice cream.

How Parents View Family Meals

Benefits

- Time for conversation and talking about the day
- Opportunity to relax and laugh
- Healthy, home-cooked food and nutritious, balanced meals
- Family relations (connect, support, and encourage)
- Time to plan activities

Challenges

- Getting help with meal planning, preparation, and cleaning up
- Picky eaters
- Quick, easy, healthful meal ideas
- Conflicts and power struggles at mealtimes

Source: Reference 45.

Food is a necessity, but feeding is an experience. Meaningful family interactions center around food. My goal for families is to know the pleasures of eating good food and being together around the table without underlying conflict. Family mealtimes should build trust and relationships. Wonderful things can happen if parents are able to put a priority on getting good food to the table and making mealtimes a satisfying event.

Plan for Positives at Meals

Eating together as a family promotes communication. It can be a time for conversations and connection. When each of you takes responsibility for helping create a nurturing mealtime, you connect more deeply as a family. Here are suggestions to make dinner together a positive experience.

- Plan the time for dinner in advance and ask each family member (when possible) to be there.
- Share or assign responsibilities for making the meal and cleaning up after the meal. A chart on the refrigerator helps avoid fights over whose turn it is.

- Start together and finish together. If a family member is late or needs to leave early, they should excuse themselves politely. Ask that such excuses be kept to a minimum. Even very young children can learn to sit politely at the table. If this is not a habit in your family, it may take some time for everyone to get used to it.
- Pass the food so that each person can serve themselves. Expect and request good manners at the table.
- Give each person a chance to tell about his or her day or something interesting that happened. Dinner is not the time to work out stressful situations.
- If there is a TV in the room where you eat, keep it turned off during the meal.
- Remember your role. Don't get involved in *how much* (if any) your child eats.
- Don't prompt, don't reward, and don't give any disapproving "looks." Just enjoy your food and the conversation.

Parents Making Changes

To help your family get on board with changes in the family mealtime, choose only one or two changes in this list to try first. Give everyone a chance to adjust before moving on to the next change.

- Set up and follow a weekly schedule of meals and snacks.
- Plan what you will serve for meals and snacks before hunger takes over you and the kids.
- Make one meal for the whole family—not special foods for each person.
- Don't have forbidden foods. Serve favorite foods often enough that they aren't a big deal.
- Try making more foods from your heritage and your family's traditions.

- Only eat at the kitchen table, breakfast counter, or dining room table.
- Clear the table or counter of distractions. Set it with flowers or a candle, so it's a pleasant place to sit together.
- Sit with your children at the table while they eat. They need you there.
- Pay attention to the people at the table, including your child.
- Turn off the TV during meals and snacks.
- Declare mealtime special by starting with a ritual, like lighting candles, saying a blessing, or recounting each person's "best" and "worst" for the day.
- Make a firm rule that mealtime is positive family time. No arguing allowed.
- Don't expect a very young child to sit at the table longer than 15 or 20 minutes.
- Show your kids how you would like them to eat and behave at the table by how you eat and interact at the table.

Planning for Success

Your role is to plan what you will serve at meals and snacks and what foods to shop for. Everyone struggles with planning meals, but planning and making sure everyone knows the schedule sure simplifies your life. To help, I have gathered some ideas in the recipe section at the end of the book. I also recommend that you scan cooking and lifestyle magazines for recipes, watch cooking shows, check cookbooks out of the library, and search for recipes on the Internet with the ingredients you want to use. The fact that you are searching will keep new ideas coming to you for ways to make simple, healthy meals.

Keep in mind that it is fine for your dinner to be "boring." If your children are hungry, they will eat. Think about it this way: If you are concerned that the folks in your family are

Sample Weekly Dinner Schedule	
Sunday	Spaghetti Pie (make 2) and salad
Monday	Mexican Chicken Soup (make double portion) and cottage cheese
Tuesday	Leftover spaghetti pie with cooked broccoli
Wednesday	Grilled hamburgers with cooked peas and salad
Thursday	Leftover soup and applesauce
Friday	Delivery pizza with salad and cooked green beans
Saturday	Grilled or baked chicken with vegetables from the farmer's market
Snacks for the week	Almonds, cantaloupe, celery sticks and peanut butter, apples, and Chex mix

overeating, what is the need to serve exciting, stimulating food? We all eat too much at buffets in part because there are so many exciting choices. Better to have "boring" Southwestern Soup, which is full of healthy vegetables every single Monday night. Then you won't have to think, and your family all get to eat a healthy dinner.

Share the Burden

⊚ Cook together with another family or friend. Two families I know alternate cooking on Mondays. One mom cooks twice the normal amount and the other family comes by to pick it up—and the next Monday they switch.

⊚ In some areas, there are places where you can go and put together healthy meals in advance that you cook at home. They even encourage having a get-together with your friends while you plan meals and assemble your items. Talk with them before you sign up to see if they will make food that will be healthy for you.

Do they use in seasonal vegetables? Are the meals high in legumes, vegetables, and whole grains? Are the fats healthy—olive oil and other unsaturated fats? Are meats and cheeses in smaller portions compared to the vegetables?

- If you have a teenager, get him or her involved. Boys and girls can be responsible for a portion of the preparation—the salad or the vegetable. Gradually, they can be responsible for several items or even the full meal. This is a win-win situation because they are learning skills, planning, and responsibility (and consequences if you don't pay attention to how long something has been cooking!) and you get to be supervisor—not the primary chef for the night.

- The cook doesn't have to clean up. This was always the rule in my house. Even very young children can clear their own plates and help put things back in the refrigerator. Older children can learn to do a good job cleaning up. Expect them to do it well, and check that they do. Don't let them get away with a half-hearted job that you just have to finish later. Put on some "cleaning up the kitchen" music and dance your way through it. No music? You all can sing, can't you?

The Challenge of the Busy Schedule

There is no magic for fitting good habits into a busy schedule. The key is to make family meals a priority, simplify what you serve, and plan meals ahead of time. The fact that you are reading this book is a good sign that you are already prioritizing your family's health. Do you struggle with a busy schedule and barely see each other at the table?

It's like this: A simple meal takes less time to prepare. A simply furnished, uncluttered room takes less time to clean. Fewer possessions mean less time to maintain them and fix them and find room for them. Fewer clothes mean less time debating which pair of jeans to wear. Simplifying is also good for the environment and the world from which we consume. One book on simplifying (*Simpler Living, Compassionate Life: A Christian Perspective;* see Resources) helped me to think about how my everyday choices combine to create the tone of my life.

It certainly helps if one parent is able to have a shorter work schedule. My mom stayed home with us when I was little. When my little brother went to first grade, my mom went back to school to get her degree. I remember, because she was in class until late, and my dad cooked dinner. He could cook

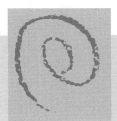

Question for the Psychologist

Q **We are starting to make some changes and now have sit-down family meals. When my brother comes over, his kids just take food and run back to the TV. Can I make them sit with us? How do I get my brother to control his kids at my house?**

A First, I want to praise you for your good management: you won your family's cooperation to have sit-down family meals. Use some of that good management on your brother. Call and ask if he would be willing to support your efforts for your family by telling his kids that at your place they are required to eat at the table. When it's time to serve the food, give a reminder, such as: "Remember, at our house everyone stays at the table to eat their food." Turn the TV off. If one of the kids takes his food away from the table, ask him individually and quietly to come back to the table, because that is the rule at your house. That is about all you can do. If you still do not get cooperation, you have a choice: tell your kids they must follow the rules even when their cousins don't or tell your brother that he and his kids are not welcome for meals until he can get them to cooperate.

ground beef 10 different ways. (I am pretty sure that is why I learned to cook at the age of 8—self-preservation.) The great thing was that my dad was able to arrange his schedule to be home right after we got home from school. He supervised us in helping with dinner, eating, and cleaning up. I can't remember ever going to a restaurant unless we were traveling. I know my dad had to work more at night and on the weekends because of this schedule, but I also know that having a home-cooked meal and eating together were really important for us as a family and as individuals.

Eating Out: The "Quick" Myth

Many times when we are busy, we seek a "faster" solution instead of the simpler one. Does eating out or getting take-out food seem faster than making dinner? Consider the extra driving to get there, and the time spent waiting in line for the food. Faster is not healthier, and it's not always really faster either. Raising a healthy child requires time, thought, and some work, too. You have choices to make.

- Plan what to serve for meals and snacks for the week, and write a shopping list to start the week off right.
- Use "quick meals" cookbooks and meal planners to help you. The library and Internet have many to choose from.
- Prepare some parts of the meal ahead of time—that only need warming to serve.
- Plan for leftovers (you can make a big pot of soup on the weekend) for the days you know you'll get home late.
- Don't stop on the way home. Teach your children that it's okay to be hungry for a few more minutes.
- Everyone is cranky when they are hungry. Set out a few nuts, cheese slices, or whole wheat crackers while you heat up dinner. Put something on a plate for everyone to share rather than putting out the whole box.

◎ Keep a list of snack suggestions on the pantry door for easy ideas at snack time.

◎ Save a plate of food for a family member who will be late so they don't have to eat out.

Tips for Saving Time Making Meals

◎ When you have time to make a dish, make two and freeze one. This works well for dishes like lasagnas or casseroles.

◎ If possible, have a separate freezer. Most freezer compartments in refrigerators do not stay consistently cold enough, which can damage the food and over time it will get "freezer burn."

◎ Go to the farmer's market and buy what is in season and plentiful. You can freeze foods in easily usable quantities. You are imitating what you find at the supermarket, but you make it yourself and know the quality better.

Eating at Home Is Healthier

Eating at home gives you control over what is in the food. Food prepared at home typically does not have as much sugar or fat as restaurant food. The goal at the restaurants is *not* your child's long-term health; it's to get you to buy the food, eat more of it, and return again and again.

Eating at home decreases the choices: there is no 30-item menu. "All you can eat" buffets are a well-known way to interfere with your inner knowing that you are full. When you can take as much as you want with lots of choices, it's easy to go overboard. All-you-can-eat cafeterias contribute to the common weight gain of teens who go off to college. Most people overeat when they can choose from many different foods. Think

> Create a new family habit of eating food from a restaurant only once a week or less.

about holiday meals, when we fill the table with so many good foods and leave the table groaning about "too much." Family dinners at home have much more limited choices and do not present the temptation to overeat. Remember that another of your roles as a parent is to decide what menu items are allowed for ordering when your family eats out.

Eating at home allows you and your children more choice on the size of the servings. How much a child eats is his or her responsibility. You don't have to worry about how much they eat. It's good to be aware that many restaurant meals come in portions that are way too large. When you order an entrée at a restaurant, it has to be big enough to satisfy almost everyone who would order it—otherwise, some customers would feel they weren't getting enough for their money and not eat there again. When you eat out, you can ask for a "take home box" first and put half the entrée into it before you eat the other half—or you can share it with another family member. You don't have to eat it all. Large portions encourage everyone to overeat.

When Your Child Won't Eat at Mealtimes

Sometimes, you will sit down to eat together, but your child will not eat. Then 5 minutes after dinner is over, he or she is back and asking for food. This is one of the reasons that you need a meal schedule. You and your child need to be able to know when food will be eaten. If you allow children to eat randomly, they will learn that they don't have to eat at dinner—they can eat whenever. Stick to your schedule.

A later chapter on picky eaters includes the story of Annie. She tried this on her mom but Catherine had a consistent approach. When Annie returned complaining of hunger, Catherine got her plate out of the refrigerator and helped her sit back down at the table for dinner try number 2. Annie soon learned that the food choices wouldn't change later—it was still the same dinner—and this behavior soon stopped.

  ◎ Don't nag, bribe, prompt, or shame.
  ◎ Don't play games to encourage your child to eat.

- ⊚ Children will want to eat because they see you eating.
- ⊚ Don't pressure your child to eat "for me" or any other reason.
- ⊚ Remind them to eat at snack time—then put it away after 15 minutes or so.
- ⊚ Define where food is eaten in your house—and set limits on eating outside those areas.

If you are having trouble getting your family to eat together, think a little about what else might be going on. Is the atmosphere too chaotic for your child to focus on eating? Have you turned off the TV and radio? Do you give notice that it's almost dinnertime—to give your child some preparation time? Try having a pre-dinner ritual, like always going to the bathroom to wash up for dinner. This physical activity will help your child learn the routine of when you eat. Is the afternoon snack too close to dinnertime, and she just isn't hungry? As much as you can, be consistent about when you eat, because our bodies run on an internal clock influenced by night and day. Children function best on a consistent schedule.

Where Does Dessert Fit In?

Dessert is just one part of the meal. It shouldn't be a reward for finishing or overeating other food. The end of dinner is a good time for sweet foods. It's hard to overeat something sweet if your child has already eaten reasonable amounts of dinner.

Some kids do try to play games by being "not hungry" for the broccoli, pork chops, and potatoes but suddenly become hungry for the cranberry cake and ice cream. It's not the end of the world if all your child eats is the cake and ice cream. In fact, if you made a whole wheat cranberry cake to add to the calcium and protein in the ice cream, this dessert is pretty healthy. For this to happen once in a while would be fine. But if this is the pattern for your child (avoiding the dinner food and only eating dessert), stop serving dessert for a few weeks. This will him or her realize that the dinner foods are tasty and a good way to fill up.

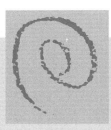

Question for the Psychologist

Q**How do I get my teenager to sit at the table with us?**

A Use small steps, irresistible invitations, respectful requests, and logical consequences. Teenagers quickly become set in their ways, think they are big enough to refuse, and have a million things they would rather do than converse with you while eating. Start with a minimal plan such as dinner together twice a week, with no more than 30 minutes sit-down time required. Plan menus that please your teen, but do not expect or demand compliments or gratitude—you can promote that later. Ask sweetly; think of it as inviting a friend for dinner—no guilt trip, no threats, no whining. You may still get no for an answer. That's when you tell your teenager that you are serious about having dinner together and that if he or she will not cooperate with you, there will be a negative consequence. You need to pick a consequence that fits in your situation and is likely to persuade your teen, such as no going out that evening because you did not see enough of him or her during dinner, having to do a chore with you for alternative together time, removal of entertainment equipment from their room to make it less competitive with family dinner time, or loss of phone privileges for a day or two to give them more time for family dinner invitations.

14

Helping the Picky Eater

"Annie's really tough" said her mom Catherine as she was getting dinner together. "There are just a few things she will eat, so we just focus on getting a variety of things into her over time." Catherine had made chili, spaghetti noodles, and spinach for dinner and she was preparing plates for each of us. She put the noodles and some butter and lots of cheese into Annie's bowl and then put some chili on the side. "She won't eat any of the chili, but I'll put it in there anyway." said Catherine to me. As we sat down, Annie complained, "Why is there chili in my bowl?"

Catherine said, "You have noodles, too. Just eat around it." Over the course of our dinner together, Annie ate some of the noodles (which had a little chili on it, of course) and drank some milk but didn't eat the chili. When dinner ended, most of her food was still in the bowl but that didn't seem to faze Catherine or Annie's dad Samuel at all. They cleaned up the dinner dishes after the kids cleared their plates, and we all moved on to talking and looking at pictures.

Annie is definitely a picky eater. If you ask Catherine and Samuel, they can give you the short list of foods that Annie will eat. But they have developed an approach over time that uses a lot of the main principles we recommend for children. First, they expose Annie to foods that Annie won't eat and also serve her things that they know Annie likes—the noodles, cheese, and butter. The lack of pressure is perfect.[46] This will give Annie the space to try things like chili eventually when she decides she is ready. And, Catherine is also right that over time Annie will get what she needs. Today, she ate some eggs. Yesterday, the whole-wheat pasta. Tomorrow, some green beans. Each day she gets different nutrients and over a week it equals a balanced diet. Annie is petite, and she doesn't need that many calories—in fact, the few bites of pasta with cheese was probably all she needed.

As I explained in Chapter 3, children grow in spurts. So, some days they will eat more than others. Some days they are more active and need more calories. Catherine knows that Annie will eat when she is hungry.

If your child persistently doesn't eat at dinner time, think about what he or she is getting in the hours before dinner. Is the snack time too close to dinner? Does he drink something that fulfills his need for calories like juice or milk in the hours before dinner? Does she drink a lot of calories at school or daycare? If your child is hungry, he or she will eat.

Tips from Parents for Dealing with Picky Eaters

- The dinner table is not a restaurant or a battlefield.
- Don't get emotional about whether your child eats or not. If you want it, they won't want it.

- If you feel yourself losing your temper, get up and take a break. Introducing a battle at dinner is just as unhelpful as unhealthy food.
- Try to focus on something else rather than what the child is eating.
- When other children come over to your house and say what foods they do and do not like, do what Catherine does and remind them that, "This is not a restaurant. This is what I am offering."
- Don't use "how many bites do I eat" to get dessert.
- Put the food out that you want them to eat.
- Everyone sits at the table until everyone is done, and then everyone eats dessert together.
- Dessert is not necessary; sometimes there is no dessert.

How Taste Develops

Have you ever been traveling and been offered something unfamiliar to eat and thought, "How can they eat that?" Children and adults alike often greet new flavors and foods with dislike. Children especially are programmed to prefer sweet and salty tastes and familiar foods. Human breast milk is sweet, although the amount of sweetness varies from mother to mother. Taste and smell are important tools to help us seek out foods that are beneficial to our bodies and to reject food that is harmful.[47] It is thought that this rejection of the unfamiliar and of bitter tastes evolved, at least in part, to protect our young from eating poisons. (Although if you have ever had a newly mobile 1-year-old eat the potting soil or try to chew on the sole of your muddy boot, you know that this isn't completely effective.)

How does an infant know what to eat? Inside the womb, babies are surrounded by amniotic fluid, and, in a sense, this is the first food that an infant experiences as it swallows the fluid. Both amniotic fluid and breast milk, the next food supplied by the mother, are flavored by the diet of the mother.

Studies of infant animals help us understand how our infants know what to eat. Infant pigs actively seek and prefer the flavors of the food eaten by their mothers during pregnancy and while breastfeeding. The young animals prefer the diet of their mothers because it's familiar to them. After being weaned, a young animal must learn to eat and forage on its own and naturally is drawn to the safe foods of the mother that it has been "programmed" to like from tasting them in the womb or through breastfeeding.

Does this same imprinting occur in humans? Human infants begin swallowing amniotic fluid near the end of the third month of gestation. The amniotic fluid changes as a result of the mother's diet and probably other factors. Dr. Julie Mennella led research to look at the effect of diet.[48] She assigned pregnant women to one of three different groups. Group 1 drank carrot juice several times a week during the third trimester of pregnancy but did not eat or drink any carrots after starting to breastfeed. Group 2 did not have carrots until after delivery and drank carrot juice while breastfeeding. Group 3 did not eat or drink any carrots. At 6 months after birth, the mothers all introduced cereal mixed with carrot juice to their babies, and the reaction of the infants was videotaped. The babies from groups 1 and 2 had "fewer negative expressions" and their mothers perceived that their babies liked the carrot-flavored cereal better than the plain cereal. "Fewer negative expressions" is researcher language for: they liked it. The fact that this study (and others like it) have to use "fewer negative expressions" as a conclusion tells us something about infants in general: they are not going to look at us and say, "I like that!"

So, it is likely that human infants also learn important information about what is good to eat through clues in the amniotic fluid. The next food that most infants experience is breast milk. Dr. Mennella and other researchers think it may serve as a bridge between in utero flavors and the flavors in the infant's solid food, because breast milk is also flavored by the mother's diet. The infant can taste garlic, spices, beverages, tobacco, and all kinds of flavors, good and bad, in the breast milk. Your amniotic fluid and your breast milk are your baby's first exposure to the wide variety of flavors in the world and to your traditions and culture.

Your Baby's Likes and Dislikes

Babies don't really know what they like or dislike yet. They operate on familiar versus unfamiliar, and as was pointed out above, that often depends on what mom ate during pregnancy and breastfeeding. Even without being exposed to a variety of vegetables from the amniotic fluid and breast milk, your baby can learn to eat what you feed her.

Feed your baby green beans at least 10 times before even considering whether to give up. Don't pay so much attention to her facial expressions; focus more on whether she will continue to let you give her bites of it.[49] Let her play with her food, too. By around 10 months of age, babies can "explore" their food. It's a good way to get familiar with green beans. You can put some mashed up green beans in a plastic bowl and let your baby play with it during dinner.

Tips for Introducing New Foods

- When it's time to begin solid foods (around 6 months), introduce only one new food at a time over a period of several weeks to give your baby a chance to get used to the new texture and flavor.
- Introduce vegetables before fruits.
- At 8 to 9 months, babies enjoy playing with finger foods. Be sure to mash up foods into small pieces. Also, don't give them anything that would be small or firm enough to cause choking, such as raisins, peanuts, or candies.

Your Child's Likes and Dislikes

Don't overindulge your child's food preferences. Ellyn Satter puts it this way: Be considerate with meals.[50] She suggests that you have four to five items per meal. For example, serve a starch, a meat, a vegetable, a drink, and a high-fat condiment like butter, salad dressing, or gravy. Try to have at least one item that you know each person will eat. Almost everyone likes bread and butter, so bread and butter could be on the table at every meal. If one of the eaters didn't like anything else, they could just fill up on bread and butter. This means your picky eater can be exposed to a good variety of foods but also be satisfied and full at the end of the meal.

This type of approach is much better than being the "short-order cook" and leaving the table to cook different items for different family members. Don't be a short-order cook. Your family can eat the same healthy foods together.

Here are some suggestions for helping you and your child enjoy mealtimes more.

⌾ **Get your child involved.**

Annie helped Catherine bake bread last weekend, and of course, she ate a big slice when it was done. Involve the kids in the process of preparing things you like. "Watching is helping," says 6-year-old Annie, and "doing the parts that you can do is helping, too."

⌾ **Be understanding of the day-to-day variations.**

Catherine explains: "Sometimes Annie is just exhausted because we got back late from traveling or something. Then I know to expect problems. If she leaves the table without eating, I put the plate in the refrigerator and when she comes back, I warm up the food and set it out again for her. We don't really have this problem much anymore, because Annie knows what to expect. She knows that our kitchen is not a buffet. We all sit together until everybody is done eating what they want to eat. If she only eats a quarter of a sandwich, I am just relying on the fact that that is all she needed. She will eat what she needs at the next healthy snack or meal."

Try not serving things too hot or too cold.

Ice water is not as easy for children to drink as water at room temperature. Don't start with soup or casseroles scalding hot because then they have to wait and blow on it and may fool around rather than start eating right away.

Take them to the farmer's market.

Karen's children are now teenagers. When they were in early grade school, they didn't want to eat any vegetables. So she took them down to the farmer's market one Saturday morning, and they picked out the funniest looking vegetables from the big piles on the tables. She said that was it—from then on they ate vegetables.

Grow your own.

My sister Jolene has a garden behind the house, about 5 by 20 feet long. She grows tomatoes, squash, beans, herbs, and sunflowers. She said that Alice, her quite particular daughter, asks about the garden all winter. "Mommy, are you going to grow beans again?" She assures Alice that she will. The kids have strong preferences: Julian, the older brother, likes the green beans raw right off the vine, but Alice only likes them cooked. The children feel invested in the vegetables that come from the garden, which makes it much easier to serve them at the table. Growing something is a great way to interest your child in vegetables. If you don't have a spot at your house, look for a community garden and go check it out. Walk over there if you can—to start another great habit.

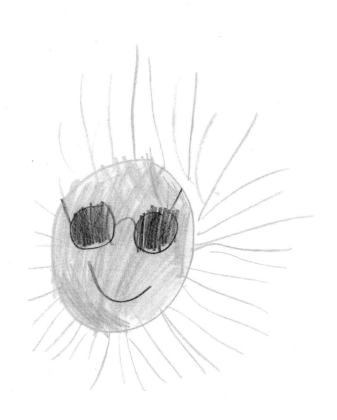

15

Good Parenting and Cooperative Children

By Cornelia Vanderkooy-Vos, PhD

To be able to make the important changes I've presented in this book in your own family, it will help to have a cooperative child. It requires respect and cooperation from your child to make many of the changes you want to make. I am often confronted by clear examples of ineffective parenting in my clinic. These are parents who, for whatever reason, are failing. This situation can be turned around, and to help you, I sought the wisdom of my favorite psychologist, my mother, Dr. Cornelia Vanderkooy-Vos, who wrote the following chapter and answered the "Questions for the Psychologist" throughout the book.

There is no magic wand for parents. You need to combine kindness with firmness. And patience! Still, getting children to cooperate with new food policies does not have to be difficult. As discussed in earlier chapters, children have a natural desire from birth to satisfy their bodies by eating, and they have a natural ability to regulate how much and what they eat. Successful parenting takes advantage of this ability. Sometimes, mistaken parenting interferes with this process.

Getting children to cooperate with changes in the family routine is no different from other tasks—whether it is food, sleep, neatness, or homework. I have learned what works from parents raising confident and responsible children—and from raising my own five children. I have boiled down what I learned into twelve tips for parents.

You may also find information and support in some of the books listed in the Resources section or from a friend or a counselor. Good parenting takes motivation, information, patience, and persistence.

⊚ **Treat your child with respect at all times.**

This is the most important tip. My *Merriam Webster Collegiate Dictionary* defines "respect" as "to consider worthy of high regard," and "to refrain from interfering with." Our children are individuals; they are separate from our selves. They have been entrusted to our care until they are able to take care of themselves. However small, they respond much better if they are approached with respect, just like you and I. Respectful treatment is kind, polite, and attentive. There is no physical harm or verbal attack, no name-calling, put-downs, shaming, accusations starting with "you never" or "you always," nor raised voices. It is best to talk to our children the way we want them to talk to us and the way we talk to our friends. Respectful treatment is not only kinder, but it is the only way to win cooperation. If you are not respectful of your children, can you expect them to be respectful of you?

◎ **Show unconditional love to your child.**

No matter how frustrating, how disappointing, how aggravating, this is still *your* child. She is unique, with gifts and flaws, and she needs to be told that you will always love her, no matter what. Don't be discouraged by your own flaws in this area; no parent succeeds in consistently showing unconditional love to her child. But, the more you succeed, the better off your child is and the more likely your child will work with you.

◎ **Be in charge.**

Do not forget, and don't let your child forget, that you are in charge. As the parent, it is your responsibility to decide what choices to give your child, and what consequences will result when he makes poor choices. Although you may make mistakes, you know more about the world than your child does. You are his teacher. Allowing a child the right degree of independence for his stage of development is a delicate matter. You do not want to be too permissive or too controlling. This takes patience and wisdom. Children have always challenged their parents' authority. Be calm and firm.

◎ **Listen to your child.**

Do your best to listen quietly and try to understand your child's viewpoint, thoughts, and feelings about a problem. There is no threat to your authority in hearing the child's point of view. Because he is an individual separate from you, it is important to know his needs and desires. This is good for your child and helps you make better decisions for your child. This interaction may motivate your child to cooperate more fully.

◎ **Understand your child's misbehavior.**

A misbehaving child is a discouraged child.[51] He is discouraged because he feels like an outsider. Children have a strong need to belong and to experience themselves as an important member of their family. They come with a built-in desire to cooperate. Discouraged children need their parents' help to get back on track. They need understanding, encouragement, guidance, and structure to help them once again become cooperative members of the family.

◎ Avoid the debate trap.

Less is more; that is, less talking is more effective. You explain the plan to your child, listen to her objections, include her suggestions, if any, and restate the plan. There is no need to justify it or to debate. You do not always have to explain your decision, and you are not required to persuade your child. If you agree to debate, your child thinks she does not have to comply unless she loses the debate—and she's the judge. Better to repeat your decision, in the same calm tone of voice. You can pretend to be a broken record. Your child will get it, and you will save yourself a lot of words.

◎ Offer choices to your children.

We may expect our children to do as we say, but every parent knows that they can and will refuse and fight us on particular matters. This is just kids being kids. Don't insist, offer him the choice of cooperating or receiving a consequence. The consequence might be the natural one. If he does not eat the lunch mom or dad prepared, he will be very hungry by the next meal. Or the consequence might be the logical one. If the child won't clean up after preparing his snack in the way he has been shown, then he loses the privilege of preparing his own snack the next day. It is not respectful to order a child to do something, because it does not acknowledge the child as a separate, independent being. "Put your plate in the dishwasher" is not nearly as kind as "Please put your plate in the dishwasher." This approach is more likely to win your child's cooperation.

Control your emotions.

Although easier said than done, controlling your emotions is the key to staying in charge and encouraging cooperation. Of course, there are times when you will get angry at your misbehaving child. If you vent that anger on the child, you are behaving disrespectfully to him. That will cause him to lose respect for you, and he will sense that you are not in control anymore. It is better to take time to cool off and tend to your emotions. Spend some time alone, reflect on what bothered you so much, and vent your feelings to an understanding friend or counselor. Anger management involves owning the feeling, taking time to tend to the feeling, and learning to interpret the situation differently. So your fight was about Josh coming home in time for supper, but it escalated to his saying ugly things to you. The best approach is not to take it personally and to use the situation as a teaching moment. You can give him a consequence for the disrespect and a choice about supper—either come home in time or you will take his car keys for the next three days.

Be manipulation-proof.

Kids will be kids, and they will try to manipulate you into agreeing to something that is not good for them. Thomas Phelan, PhD, in his book, *1-2-3 Magic: Effective Discipline for Children 2–12*,[52] reports children's three favorite methods of manipulation.

— **Badgering** consists of endless repetition of the same request or word, such as "Please, please, please. . . ." It is useless to persuade her to stop; the best thing is to ignore her or send her to her room.

Martyrdom is designed to push mom or dad's guilt button. It takes the form of pouting, crying, or some form of inaction such as refusing to play. When you see through this one, you can cheerfully tell him that he is welcome to be unhappy as long as he wants and that you yourself see no reason to be unhappy, too.

Intimidation is an aggressive attack often involving a temper tantrum with yelling, throwing, storming, swearing, or accusations. This is designed to make you cave in. The best response is to leave the scene until the storm is over and then apply a logical consequence appropriate to the child's age for the bad behavior.

Be patient.

It takes time to train a child to do something differently. Your child may resist you at first, testing you with manipulation or just plain refusal. He is not sure you are serious unless you pass these tests. Be prepared to give him a second chance, and after that, to apply the logical consequence that you said you would do. No need to raise your voice. No need to get emotional. No need to explain the reasons more than twice at the most. Be a broken record and repeat what is expected. Stay friendly. Don't give up. Be consistent. Remember, if you give in after three times, you are coaching your child to try at least three times. Once your child realizes you are serious, and once he is getting used to the change, he will stop resisting.

Leave power struggles.

Children will try to engage parents in power struggles. It is their mistaken way to try to be somebody, to assert that they are important. It takes the form of "You cannot make me," or "You cannot stop me."

Examples are: S won't stop chewing her food with her mouth open; T refuses to eat what Mom prepared; J refuses to help with washing the dishes. In each of these examples, the parent learned the hard way that the authority figure cannot win a power struggle: the parent cannot make the child do something he refuses to do, and, after a certain age, the parent cannot stop the child from doing what he insists on doing. When parents recognize and accept that they cannot win a power struggle, they leave the conflict. By leaving the conflict, they can calm down, stop being emotional, and figure out how to regain their child's cooperation. Parents can stay in charge by using natural or logical consequences. If S insists on keeping her mouth open while chewing, you could ask her to leave the table to spare others the experience of observing her, and invite her to eat after the others are done. T may choose whether to eat what has been prepared, but you can decide that you have provided suitable food for him, and nothing else is available until the next snack or mealtime. You could give J a choice between helping with the dishes or losing all after-dinner entertainment privileges for the rest of the evening. As the parent, you give notice that in spite of the challenge to your authority, you are in charge, and you arrange it so that the benefits of cooperation outweigh the benefits of refusal.

◎ **Work around spouse problems the best you can.**
Parents often disagree about how to parent, and the area of healthy habits is no exception. First, show respect. Second, be humble: you may be going a little overboard. Talk things over, listen, and identify the truth of what the other is saying. Explain the problem as you see it. Find out how the other suggests changing things for the better, and see if you can try

it that way. Look for compromises. Try a temporary change and then renegotiate when you can weigh the benefits to your family. Try to find agreement about what you both can live with. Remember that harmony in your home is more important than how and when healthier habits are established.

None of these tips were a surprise to you. They are basically about how to get along with other people plus how to be in charge. Try to combine a loving attitude with a firm and wise approach. You will be glad you were persistent, and your children will thank you when they are parents themselves.

16

When Changes Aren't Working

Michael, a teenager, had been referred to me for weight gain, high cholesterol, and high blood pressure. At the first appointment, Michael and his mom identified several great target areas for change. He had been eating a low-fiber, high-sugar breakfast cereal. He watched many hours of TV during an average day. He frequently drank sports drinks, even when not at football practice. At his follow-up appointment 2 weeks later, after the nutritionist had seen him, she came to my desk and shook her head a little saying, "He gained more weight." It was disappointing, but that didn't tell the whole story.

The nutritionist was excited because Michael and his mom had made big changes. He was drinking more water and playing outside more. Michael told me, "Mom threw out all the junk food, the sugary cereal, the chips, the fruit punch. We just woke up, and it was gone, and there were six boxes of bran cereal sitting where all that used to be!"

I could tell he was impressed and, of course, a little shocked and perhaps a little proud that his mom cared enough about him to make those changes. Jennifer and I were so proud of both of them. Michael's weight gain was much less important than these new healthy changes, and the changes were the focus of the visit. I know that Michael will still eat some "junk food" and he will still drink some sport drinks. But there will be less of them, and over time he will be healthier for it—and his weight will come back into balance.

Measuring Success

Do children ever just keep gaining weight, even if you make all these changes? Sometimes, yes. But realize that success can be measured in many ways: improved physical fitness, stable eating patterns and nurturing mealtimes, more vegetables in your meals, and fewer chronic diseases now and 20 years from now. These are all signs of success, even without weight loss. Staying at the same weight is a great accomplishment. As children grow taller, that weight will fit them better.

Family Dynamics

I have seen families where positive lifestyle changes weren't possible. Sometimes a teenager won't make changes and eats and drinks enough outside the home to continue to gain weight. In this case, I advise parents to change what they can. Restricting foods or food fights don't work. Continue to provide healthy food at home, and have faith that, eventually, these positive actions will pay off.

Another challenge can be your own issues. Sometimes mom or dad, or both, have their own complicated issues and are not able to really commit to these healthy changes. Sometimes you have to become the parent *you* never had. Working through your own feelings and issues is critical because our children are extremely savvy at seeing us as we really are.

I had been seeing 15-year-old Belinda and her mom for almost a year, but each time she came in, they had not been able to make sustainable changes. Belinda had lots of gastro-intestinal complaints—abdominal pain, diarrhea—as well as chest pain and fatigue. She was 278 pounds and gaining. While in my office, Belinda would report that everything was fine: she was walking and drinking water. But Belinda's mom would tell me a different tale, and she was very distressed about Belinda's health. At the first visit, the mother had been worried that cancer might be causing all of Belinda's symptoms. But we were able to resolve Belinda's abdominal pain, diarrhea, and chest pain, and she didn't have cancer. Each time they returned, Belinda had a new health problem. She was missing lots of school and forcing her mom to miss work. Often, she would be "sick" early in the morning and miss the school bus but would be fine several hours later. Her mother would miss several hours of work to take care of Belinda in the morning and then drive her to school. Gradually, it became clear that this family had a complicated situation. Belinda's mother felt guilty about taking her away from her father when she divorced him, so she didn't want to be too hard on Belinda. Belinda had some anger toward her mother about this as well, and she was a typical teenager, taking advantage of whatever she could. Belinda was manipulating her mother.

A situation like this requires the help of a therapist. If there are significant emotional issues in your home, adding power struggles over soda, TV time, and so forth is the last thing you need. During this year, I have seen Belinda's mom start to identify more of her own emotions, and she attends a support group. She decided to focus more on healthy habits for herself and less on what she can and can't get Belinda to do. She is becoming a positive role model. I can't predict what will happen to Belinda's health in the future, but I am very hopeful that she will follow her mom's lead.

Finding Outside Help

Sometimes your child's weight problem is not something you can tackle on your own. If your child is very overweight and especially if he or she is already a teenager and has stopped growing taller (which makes it harder to lose weight), consider having your child join a program designed for children or teens. Ask your pediatrician about lifestyle-change programs in your community. Find parents who have participated in the program and find out what they liked and disliked about it.

A worthwhile program will

- Emphasize long-term changes—not short-term dieting!
- Emphasize increasing daily physical activity
- Have a positive approach, supporting and enhancing the child's sense of self-worth no matter what they weigh
- Offer families frequent visits at first and then fewer over time but allow you to come back for support and "maintenance" over the long term

A weight treatment program can help you problem-solve and motivate you and your child. Remember, even if you are in a program, over the long run, the choices you and your child make every day at home and school will be most important in your success.

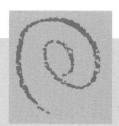

Question for the Psychologist

Q **I feel really bad about some of the things I eat. How can I tell my kids what to eat when I can't control my own eating?**

A Have you considered talking to a nutritionist or a counselor to help you understand why you make the food choices that you do? The self-knowledge you can gain from these discussions is important for your own sake. And it will help you be a better role model for your children. In the meantime, how do you decide what to offer your kids to eat? First of all, don't expect yourself to be perfect. You are wise to try to avoid giving them a double standard. Can you ask them to help you plan and prepare some meals? Could you schedule family outings to burn off some extra calories? This could be the time to get everyone thinking about how far you need to walk to burn off a doughnut or a bag of chips, for example. You might plan a time once a week when everyone gets to eat as much as they want of a special item. That might help satisfy your cravings and would not be that big a deal for everyone's health. Remember, the family has to make one change at a time—and it works best when you all make the changes together.

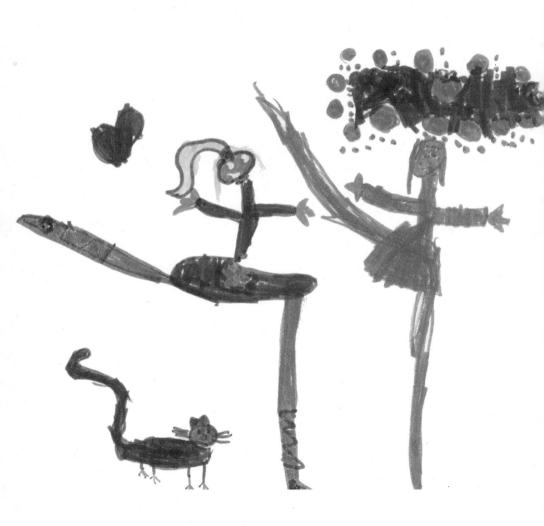

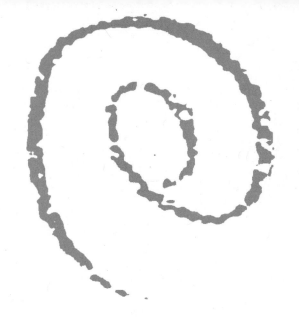

Your Child's
Nutrition Needs

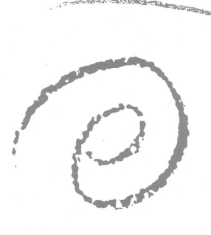

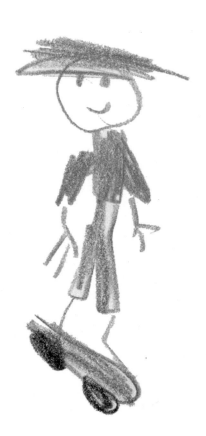

17

Nutrition ABCs and Reading the Food Label

What do our bodies need? Basically, our bodies need air, water, and food. From the food we eat, our bodies get energy and building materials. When you think about it, it is pretty amazing that the bread, carrots, squash, and chicken we eat every day get made into all the different cells and tissues of our bodies. Using the nutrients from our food, our body remakes the cells in every tissue— a constant body remodeling. The building blocks are macronutrients: carbohydrates, protein, and fats. Micronutrients like vitamins and minerals are the helpers that make the remodeling reactions in cells go forward.

The other amazing thing about our bodies is that we can eat a seemingly random selection of food and usually end up with mostly what we need in the short term. I commonly measure nutrient levels in my patients, and only rarely do I find nutrition deficiencies in children. That said, I do think that there are a lot of important changes that result from an "unhealthy" diet that are not measurable in the short term. Those changes happen over the years and result in the chronic diseases that you are familiar with, like heart disease, diabetes, hypertension, and more.

So, what is the best way to make sure that your food gives your body what it needs to be healthy? It's important to eat a variety of foods, such as carbohydrates, proteins, vegetables, fruits, and fats. By eating a variety of foods (especially vegetables), you give your body a variety of micronutrients. Eating these foods in the right proportions also helps balance your nutritional needs. To prepare you to plan meals, it's good to know some details about food.

Carbohydrates

Carbs come in three forms: starches (like potatoes and breads), sugars, and fiber.

⊜ **Starches.**

In nature, starch is combined with some fiber. A good example is wheat or rice. A kernel of wheat has a brown outer wrapping called the *bran*. This wrapping is mostly fiber plus vitamins, minerals, and a bit of healthy fat. However, when a food manufacturer makes white flour or white rice, the outer wrapping is removed, and all those nutrients are lost. Even if the manufacturer puts some vitamins back in the flour or the rice, it is not as healthy as it was before. Whole-grain flour and brown rice have it all: all the vitamins, minerals, and fiber.

Sugars.

Sugars are absorbed rapidly into the bloodstream and are a good source of quick energy. Some sugars are natural and found in milk, fruits, and vegetables. Natural sweeteners are cane sugar, beet sugar, and honey. However, many types of sugar are now added to packaged foods. These sugars have many different names. Some of the more common names for sugar on food packaging are:

- Cane sugar or sugar
- Sucrose
- Fructose
- Dextrose
- Maltose
- Lactose
- High-fructose corn syrup
- Corn syrup

Lactose is the main sugar naturally found in milk. Some people have less ability to digest lactose. The common symptoms of lactose intolerance are increased gas and diarrhea several hours after drinking milk or eating milk products.

High-fructose corn syrup is a mixture of glucose and fructose that is used in many processed foods and drinks. High-fructose corn syrup is very similar to regular (cane) sugar but it is easier to use in the manufacturing process and gives processed foods a better texture. Both sugar and high-fructose corn syrup can be harmful if they are extra calories that weren't needed. There is more information about sugars in Chapter 12.

Fiber.

Fiber is really a type of starch (carbohydrate) that our digestive system doesn't break down easily, so it passes on through without being digested.

But it makes our digestive system work better. Fiber is found in fruits, vegetables, beans, nuts, and whole grains. It adds bulk to your diet and helps prevent constipation. Eating more fiber has lots of positive effects, including making you feel better and decreasing the risk of diseases such as colon cancer, cardiovascular diseases, and diverticulitis. High-fiber foods tend to be more filling, so you feel satisfied with fewer calories.

If you decide to add more fiber to your meals and snacks, start slowly and increase it a little at a time. This allows your digestive system to adjust to the change. Increasing fiber too much too quickly can cause gas, bloating, and cramps. In the recipe section, you'll find the Breakfast Muffins (see page 226). I love these muffins, and it's very easy for me to eat two in a row when I first make them. Each muffin has a full day's requirement of fiber, so two of them can be a bit much if I haven't had them in a while. If I have only one every morning for breakfast, I adjust and don't notice any symptoms. The other important thing to know about fiber is that it needs water to work well. As you add fiber, make sure that you and your children drink plenty of water. Fiber absorbs water to make the stool soft and bulky.

Proteins

Proteins provide the building materials for all the cells in the body. The building materials are called *amino acids,* and there are 20 different ones. They are used to grow tissue and to make hormones, antibodies, and enzymes that keep the body running properly. Proteins can come from animals or plants.

Proteins from animals, such as beef, poultry, fish, dairy products, and eggs, are considered the best sources because they provide all the amino acids we need. They are called "complete" proteins because they provide the essential amino acids.

No plant proteins contain all the essential amino acids. So we have to combine two or more plant foods, such as beans and rice, to get all the amino acids we need. Plant proteins include nuts, beans and lentils, corn, soy milk, and tofu.

Beans contain six of the eight essential amino acids, and brown rice contains a different set of five amino acids. There will be some overlap, but they help each other fill any gaps that the other food might be missing. These plant food combinations can be found in any culture. In the American culture, it may be a peanut butter sandwich on whole wheat bread. In Latino cultures, it may be beans and corn tortillas. In Middle Eastern cultures, it could be lentils and rice. These combinations are a healthy substitute for meat because they are less expensive, often have less fat, and always have more fiber (meat has no fiber).

Vitamins and Minerals

Vitamins and minerals are key to every process that takes place in your body. They work in partnership with other nutrients in your food. You get vitamins and minerals from eating a wide variety of foods, in particular from eating lots of vegetables, some fruit, and some whole grains. Research shows that you can lower the risk of cancer by eating more fruits, vegetables, and grains. Vitamin supplements have not been shown to be as effective as the natural foods. (Food has always been the best medicine.) I like to eat a variety of vegetables to help make sure I get a variety of vitamins and minerals throughout the week. I also try to

---

Meal Balancing Tip

The nutrition students I know taught me one simple way to plan a meal: the plate method. Draw an imaginary line down the middle of a dinner plate and another line across it, so you have four sections of the plate to fill. One section holds the meat or protein for the meal. One section holds the potato or rice (carb) for the meal. And the other half of the plate is for the vegetables. Add a whole-grain roll and butter and a glass of milk or water, and you have a balanced dinner.

buy my vegetables when they are in season—and locally—because I know they will taste better and be more nutritious.

Finding Nutrients in Packaged Food

The food label, or Nutrition Facts panel, is very useful. Below is an example food label taken from the FDA's web article "The Food Label," located at http://www.cfsan.fda.gov/~dms/fdnewlab.html. This label will be our study tool.

Serving Size: All the information on the label is about the serving size, not the whole package. Sometimes the package only contains one serving, but more commonly there are several servings in a package.

Serving Size: ½ cup
Servings per Container: 4

In this example, *there are four servings in this container.* If your child eats the whole box, he or she has eaten four servings. The numbers on this label are for *only* the ½ cup serving—*not the whole package.*

If this were the label on a package of macaroni and cheese, a hungry teenager might easily eat the entire package in one sitting. In that case, the teen would have to multiply by four to get the number of calories for the whole package:

90 calories × 4 servings = 360 calories

That same teenager could cook some frozen broccoli along with the macaroni (and then add the cheese sauce), eat one half of the amount in the pan

---

Nutrition Facts

Serving Size 1/2 cup (114g)
Servings Per Container 4

Amount Per Serving

Calories 90   Calories from Fat 30

	% Daily Value*
Total Fat 3g	**5%**
Saturated Fat 0g	**0%**
Cholesterol 0mg	**0%**
Sodium 300mg	**13%**
Total Carbohydrate 13g	**4%**
Dietary Fiber 3g	**12%**
Sugars 3g	
Protein 3g	

Vitamin A 80%	•	Vitamin C 60%	
Calcium 4%	•	Iron 10%	

*Percent Daily Values are based on a 2,000 calorie diet. Your daily values may be higher or lower depending on your calorie needs.

		Calories: 2,000	2,500
Total Fat	Less than	65g	80g
Sat Fat	Less than	20g	25g
Cholesterol	Less than	300mg	300mg
Sodium	Less than	2,400mg	2,400mg
Total Carbohydrate		300g	375g
Dietary Fiber		25g	30g

Calories per gram:
Fat 9 • Carbohydrate 4 • Protein 4

(which is now just two servings of the mac and cheese), and combine this with a glass of milk and an apple. If he is still hungry and wants another serving of the mac and cheese, that is fine, because he has already created a balance through the variety of foods in his meal. For mac and cheese, a quick and easy way to make it healthier is to add some frozen/canned/fresh vegetables to the pasta while it's boiling. My favorite is green peas. For more tips, see the Centers for Disease Control Web site: www.cdc.gov/nccdphp/dnpa/healthyweight/healthy_eating/ energy_density.htm.

My Approach to the Nutrition Label

I tend to use the nutrition label *selectively*. If I am buying meat, potatoes, vegetables, or salad, I don't need a food label. But if I am buying a food product, particularly a new one, it can be helpful. Cereal is a good example. I prefer to have cereal that is high in fiber and not too sweet, and cereals seem to change all the time. The ingredients list gives me a clue— I can check how far down the list the sweetener is. Then I check the Nutrition Facts to see the number of grams of sugar in a serving of the cereal.

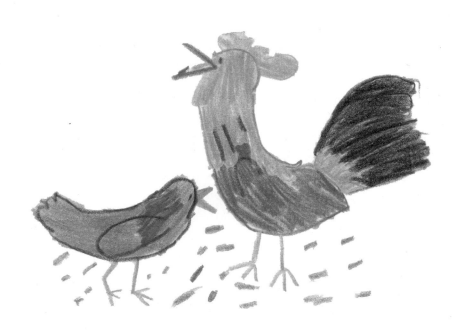

18

The Good Fats We Need to Eat

You may remember the era of "low-fat" diets, but you don't hear about them so much any more. As a nutrition researcher, I see that rush to put everyone on a low-fat diet as a lesson we don't want to repeat. Based on some early research about low-fat eating, a nutrition policy was set for the whole country. I think bad luck was involved too, because this diet took off in the minds of food manufacturers. It seems to make sense—avoid fat so you won't be fat! Special foods were created. Diets were created. Industries thrived. But people got fatter, and children got more and more overweight.

There are two main concerns behind the low-fat diet. One is that fat is the culprit for the extra calories that kids are consuming. Gram for gram, fat has more calories than carbohydrates and protein. Not only this, but foods high in fat taste extra good. Think of potato chips and fried chicken. A kid might eat more of something that tastes so delicious. The other concern is that certain fats, such as cholesterol and saturated fat, contribute to cardiovascular disease.

However, it turns out that eating fats does not automatically lead to weight gain. And keep in mind that most of the studies that demonstrated the benefits of a low-fat diet were done in middle-aged men—not children.[53]

An Extremely Low-Fat Diet Can Cause Problems

Tina's mom brought her to see me because she had elevated liver enzymes. She was just 5 years old, and the discovery that her liver numbers were high had shocked her mom. She had always been extremely particular about Tina's food. For instance, they eat only organic vegetables and dairy. In addition, she limits the meat the family eats.

After Tina's pediatrician had identified the "liver problem," Tina's mom had put her on a fat-free diet. I am not sure why Tina's mom thought there was a connection, but by the time Tina came to see me, she had been on a fat-free diet for almost 6 months. And it was a strict fat-free diet. The child in front of me was thin and pale and had a slightly wasted appearance. Her cheeks were sunken in. Tina had lost 5 pounds over the summer, and because she had started out at a normal weight, this diet clearly had not been good for her. Tina's mom told me that Tina eats all the time—as if she just can't get enough.

When we measured Tina's fat-soluble vitamins, she was low in vitamin E and vitamin D, both important for growing bodies. Clearly, she was not getting enough calories. In a healthy diet, anywhere from 25% to 35% of the calories come from eating fat; therefore, going down to almost zero is not beneficial. I counseled Tina's mom on the need for fat in Tina's diet, and started the evaluation for her elevated liver enzymes (which were not related to her low-fat diet).

At the next appointment, Tina gleefully told me, "I am drinking whole milk!" Her cheeks were now rosy, and she had gained 4 pounds back. Her mom was tossing a little olive oil with the vegetables and was allowing regular cheese and eggs again. Her mom reported that for the first few weeks of adding back fats, Tina ate around the clock, but that now she had a more typical pattern, she didn't seem to be hungry between snacks and meals. The extremes—a fat-free diet or a very high-fat diet—are just not healthy for children.

A Healthy Diet Includes Some Fat

My friends marvel at me because I use whole milk in my coffee, cook with olive oil and butter, eat nuts for snacks, and have eggs for breakfast. My favorite treat when I go out is onion rings, and I even have a mental list of which restaurants make the best ones. I make my oatmeal cookies with one cup of real, growth-hormone–free butter. If you have been following a low-fat diet, this may sound like a shocking list to you—all these fats!

First of all, our bodies need to have fats if they are going to work well. The fats that I choose are meeting my needs very well.

Second, let me tell you what else I am doing. I eat a big salad (often with avocado in it, another good source of healthy fat) and a cooked vegetable or two with the rest of my dinner or even as my dinner. For lunch, I have one or two vegetables and something with protein from the buffet. For a sweet treat, I eat dark chocolate or two homemade cookies in a day, usually as my afternoon snack and that satisfies me—there are plenty more to eat tomorrow. I often have oatmeal, granola, or some Kashi cereal for breakfast. And I have a big breakfast with eggs on the weekend. I have cheese or nuts for a snack, and I eat fresh fish whenever I can get it. My diet is a complex mix of saturated fats, unsaturated fats, monounsaturated fats, polyunsaturated fats, omega-3 and omega-6 fatty acids, plus lots of vegetables, fiber, and protein with some sugars.

This is similar to the diet I grew up with, and it's what I have available in fresh, quality forms from the markets near me. It's healthy because I feel satisfied, I have good energy, and I don't gain weight or lose weight. This way of eating provides me with a variety of fats that are just one part of a diet that matches my energy needs. I exercise a lot, and so my calorie need on a daily basis is relatively high. I can use the fats for energy. I also know from sifting through the research on these subjects that *moderation* is the key.

Fats

Fats are powerhouse foods, packing more calories per gram than protein or carbs. They keep us warm, make bodily processes work better, and taste good, too.

- Saturated fat: Animal fat, butter, coconut oil,
- Monounsaturated fat: Nuts (almonds, cashews, peanuts, and pecans), avocado, olive oil and olives, canola oil, sesame seeds, peanut butter and peanut oil, grapeseed oil, peanut oil, flaxseed oil
- Polyunsaturated fat: Corn oil, safflower oil, soybean oil, sunflower oil, walnuts, pumpkin seeds, sunflower seeds
- Omega-3 fatty acids: Walnuts, flaxseeds and flaxseed oil, canola oil, Albacore tuna, herring, mackerel, rainbow trout, sardines, salmon

Trans Fats

Trans fats are created during a process called hydrogenation that is used to turn liquid oils into solid fats. New research has shown that trans fat is probably as bad or worse than saturated fat (butter) for cardiovascular risk. Manufacturers are required to list the amount of trans fat per serving in the nutrition label. Look for none or less than 0.5 mg per serving. Some typical foods containing trans fat are processed foods (cakes, crackers, chips, and cookies), some stick margarine, shortening, and some French fries.

Keep Moderation in Mind

What I recommend (and what I do) is not low fat and not high fat. I take the middle road. This is my best suggestion for how to approach the fat question for your child. High-fat diets clearly have a lot of calories—too much for the average child who isn't that active. Most children spend a lot of time sitting in school and sitting in front of the TV. Eating lots of high-fat foods for breakfast, lunch, and dinner is a large amount of calories. It will be hard to play enough soccer or run around enough to burn all those calories. However, a very low-fat diet is not the solution, especially not for children, because this can lead to deficiencies in the healthy fats and in fat-soluble vitamins.

What does moderate fat mean? Technically it would be a diet with 30% to 40% of calories from fat. How do you accomplish that? If you eat a variety of food and avoid a few extremes—eating out frequently, serving fried food often, and buying high-fat processed snacks—your child will probably be in this range. If you want more details, visit www.mypyramid.gov and choose "My Pyramid Tracker." You can enter the foods that your child eats in a day, and it will list the total nutrients and compare that to what is recommended. It takes a little while to enter all the foods, but it's fun and helpful to see the totals at the end, and it gives you a good idea of what percentage of your child's calories in a day come from fat.

How to Include Good Fat

For most people, fat in the diet will naturally fall into place by following some simple suggestions.

⊚ Especially if there is heart disease in your family, it's good to be aware of and limit saturated fats for your family. Some ideas:
  – Consider using olive oil in recipes and for cooking at low heat. (See recipe section for suggestions.)
  – Buy less fried food.
  – Eat at home, and grill, bake, and steam your food.
  – Use 1% or 2% milk after age 2 years.
  – Serve red meat and high-fat meat (like sausage) in small (3-ounce portions) with big helpings of vegetables, salads, and brown rice.
  – Make your own hamburgers with lean ground beef or turkey (3 ounces of cooked meat per burger) on a whole wheat bun.

⊚ Even if you don't have heart disease in your family, vary your diet and include a variety of fats in moderation.

⊚ For everyone, deep-fat fried foods are not healthy if you have them too often, so eat them once a week or less.

⊚ Don't bother with the fat-free products for children—most of these have long lists of chemicals and additives to "replace" the fat. Instead, eat more foods naturally low in fat like vegetables, fruits, legumes, and whole grains.

⊚ Vary the types of fat that are included in your diet. Try to include foods from lots of categories.

⊚ Serve smaller amounts of high-fat foods along with lots of vegetables and fruits and whole grains. In other words—eat a well-balanced diet.

Fats from vegetables, nuts, and seeds are better for you and are also very satisfying. Examples are avocados, cashews, peanuts, pumpkin seeds, and flax seeds. A small amount of fat naturally occurs in whole grains, too.

You can get less fat naturally by eating a small to moderate serving of meat. The recommended serving of meat for an adult is 3 ounces, not a quarter-pound (4-ounce) or a half-pound (8-ounce). When buying meat, multiply the number of people who will be eating by 3 ounces, and use that number to help you buy the right amount. This will save you money and help you balance the meal.

What Patients and Families Ask About Eating Fat

Isn't butter bad?

I was at dinner at a nice restaurant with some colleagues not long ago, and as the rolls were passed, I helped myself to one and a piece of what I thought was butter. Across the table, a well-respected nutritionist picked up the little package and closely examined it. "Is this butter?" she asked, squinting at the label a bit trying to see the tiny writing. It was in fact butter, to my relief and her dismay. She couldn't believe that fine restaurants were still serving butter when they should have switched to soft margarine—because butter is saturated fat. There were some students at the table with us, and I think it was confusing—two experts—and two opinions on butter. I say it's fine in small quantities as part of a balanced diet. The other expert says it's unhealthy. The bottom line is this: there is not enough evidence to say what is "right" on every little thing.

For children, there is an extra issue that may not be as important for someone who is older. My concern with feeding children artificial food products (like margarine) is that they have not been studied in children nor studied over the long term. When a new food product is invented, the ingredients are tested and approved—but it's not a 20- or 40-year study. If you learned to like margarine as a child, you may be like my dad, who still prefers it over butter. Sometimes, we find out many years later that the ingredient that made the new version of the food possible isn't that great either—like trans fat.

What about eggs?

When I was growing up, eggs were a great way to start the day, full of protein and vitamins, fast, and easy to cook. Now, my mom carefully limits herself to one or two per week and when her latest cholesterol came back slightly high she questioned whether it was still too many. I assured her it wasn't. Eggs have more monounsaturated fat than saturated fat and are a good source of vitamin E. But they have some cholesterol, which is "bad." Confusing isn't it? What to do? Eat eggs in moderation.

The concern over eggs developed because of their cholesterol content. For adults, the American Heart Association doesn't specifically limit egg consumption (www.americanheart.org). But they do recommend eating 300 mg of dietary cholesterol or less per day. Because one egg has 200 mg of cholesterol, they seem like an easy place to reduce cholesterol. But for your child, remember that eggs are one source of protein, fat, and vitamins. One egg (or less) per day is a reasonable part of a balanced diet. And because they have both protein and fat, an egg with some toast and milk can be a great way to start the day and help keep your child from being hungry between breakfast and lunch. When I am not collecting them from my own coop, I prefer to buy eggs collected from cage-free hens because I like my eggs to come from animals that have been treated humanely.

French fries?

I certainly cannot think of any health benefits of French fries . . . but I do know that most children and adults love them. So have fries sometimes, but not often, and get the small size or share a larger one between several family members. Make it a limited-occasion food, like when you are traveling or on vacation.

One easy-to-make at home version of French fries can use white or sweet potatoes. You can mix them with olive oil and bake them in the oven in 20 minutes and have a lot more nutrients than the kind from the fast food restaurants. (See Focus on Vegetables on page 233 for easy home-made fries.)

Is milk bad or good?

Neither. Milk is a our first food and for some cultures is an important part of the diet for life. But other cultures have little access to cows and don't use any dairy products in their diet. I am Dutch, so my family is from a country rich with cheese-making heritage. In Holland, my Opa and Oma (the Dutch names for grandparents) were cheese farmers. After they immigrated to Canada, they bought their own land and set up a profitable dairy farm. They sold the milk to a milk cooperative, and when I visited in the summers, I remember the big tanker truck pulling up in the yard to take the milk away. Milk and dairy products such as butter, cheese, and yogurt are important parts of my diet. For me, it's a healthy source of calories because milk is part of my balanced diet. I have colleagues from different backgrounds who eat a balanced diet with almost no dairy—and they are just as healthy.

In the United States, milk consumption has decreased, especially among children. (Review the figure on page 115 in Chapter 9.) This is worrisome because dairy has been an easy source of high-quality nutrients. And if it's being substituted by sugar-sweetened beverages, these nutrients are not being replaced. Diary has magnesium, calcium, and phosphorus and may have antioxidant properties. The reduction in consumption may be partly due to the concerns about dairy fat. If you currently serve whole milk, changing to 2% milk is an easy way to reduce some calories. Fat-

Comparing Milk—What's in One Cup?					
Type of Milk	**Calories**	**Fat (grams)**	**Protein (grams)**	**Sugar (grams)**	**Calcium (mg)**
Whole milk	146	**8**	8	13	276
2% milk	122	4.8	8	12	285
1% milk	102	2.4	8	13	285
Fat-free milk	83	0	8	13	306
Low-fat chocolate	**190**	4.8	8	**24**	272

Source: www.nal.usda.gov/fnic/foodcomp/search/index.html. Accessed April 28, 2008.

free, 1%, 2%, whole milk, and flavored milk all have the same amount of other nutrients like protein, calcium, and added vitamin D. But whole milk has the most fat, and flavored milks have the most sugar (see chart). In fact, flavored low-fat milk has the most calories per cup—making it the worst choice if you are concerned about too many calories. For most children, choosing either 1%, 2%, or fat-free milk is better.

Tips on Milk

◎ Until the age of 2, use whole milk.

◎ After age 2 years, 1% and 2% milk is fine for most children and has fewer calories per cup than whole milk.

◎ Children will get used to "plain" milk if it is what is offered; don't use strawberry or chocolate flavoring to get them to drink more. The extra calories from the added sugar sweetener are just as unnecessary as the extra calories from the fat in whole milk would have been. If they don't want milk, let them drink water.

⊚ If your child has a very low dairy intake, talk with your pediatrician to make sure that he or she is getting enough calcium and vitamin D from other sources.

⊚ Most children can use 3 cups a day of milk as part of a healthy balanced diet.

Calcium to Grow On

In the United States, dairy foods have traditionally been an important source of calcium for children.[54] Over the past several decades, the trend has been for children to drink less milk and more soda. One of the consequences of this has been that children don't get enough calcium, especially children 9 to 18 years old. Children need calcium for good bone growth, so this trend is worrisome.

Children are growing, and it is during adolescence that bones reach their "peak" or point of highest density. Having good bone mass in childhood is the best way to avoid osteoporosis, a disease of thin bones, in later life. Dairy is not the only place to get calcium (see chart), and other factors are involved in bone growth as well. The more running and jumping, the better the bone growth.

Using calcium also requires vitamin D for absorption and for utilization. Vitamin D deficiency used to be common in the 1900s but became rare after dairy products were supplemented with vitamin D. Recent studies have suggested that although

---

Calcium Requirements for Children

1 to 3 years old	500 mg/day = 2 cups of milk
4 to 8 years old	800 mg/day = 3 cups of milk
9 to 18 years old	1,300 mg/day = 4–5 cups of milk

Source: American Academy of Pediatrics Committee on Nutrition: Calcium requirements of infants, children, and adolescents. aapolicy.aapublications.org/cgi/content/full/pediatrics;104/5/1152. Accessed January 16, 2009.

Nondairy Calcium Sources

Tofu, 150 grams	347 mg
White beans, 3/4 cup	119 mg
Navy beans, 3/4 cup	93 mg
Pinto beans, 3/4 cup	53 mg
Tahini, 2 Tbsp	130 mg
Almonds, 1/4 cup	93 mg
Salmon, canned with bones, 3 oz	188 mg
Collards, 1 cup	266 mg
Spinach, 1 cup	245 mg
Rhubarb, 1 cup	348 mg
Soy beans (edamame), 1 cup	261 mg
Kale, 1 cup	179 mg
Okra, 1 cup	177 mg
Chinese cabbage (pak-choi or bok-choi), 1 cup	158 mg
Greens: turnip, beet, dandelion, 1 cup	~150 mg

Sources: www.bchealthguide.org/healthfiles/hfile68e.stm#hf005, and www.nal.usda.gov/fnic/foodcomp/Data/SR20/nutrlist/sr20w301.pdf. Accessed April 28, 2008.

complete deficiency is rare, many children don't get quite enough vitamin D anymore.[55] Vitamin D is a unique vitamin because our body makes it if our skin is exposed to sunshine. Five to fifteen minutes of sun exposure a day during the spring, summer, and fall (with a sunscreen of SPF 8 or less) will provide adequate vitamin D. It's not found naturally in many foods but some fatty fish (such as mackerel) provide it. Therefore, many foods, especially milk, are fortified with vitamin D and are a primary source for getting it during the winter.

You can see from this list that your non–milk-drinking 12-year-old would have to eat a lot of spinach and beans to get all his or her calcium! Fortified drinks like rice beverages and juice can also help but can have a lot of sugar added. If your child does not consume any dairy, cook lots of healthy greens, beans, and tofu. Talk with your pediatrician about whether your child is getting enough calcium.

19

Veggies Are
Mealtime VIPs

Vegetables are so important! They provide vitamins and micronutrients, fiber, taste, and flavor to meals and snacks. If you are like most families I see, you already know it's important to "eat your vegetables," and you are already trying, but you might have run into some stumbling blocks.

Lead by Example

The strongest predictor of which vegetables and fruits your child eats is which ones you eat.[56] Think about the list of foods that you enjoy. Some are probably healthier than others. What do you enjoy that you know is healthy? A particular fruit? A certain vegetable? A tall glass of cold water after a long walk? Serve the vegetables that *you* like for dinner. Start with this.

In general, I find that most families already eat some healthy things as well as some less healthy things. It's a matter of changing ratios and improving the balance. Also, you have to make sure that your child isn't managing to avoid healthy foods entirely. Mark came to clinic with his grandmother. They live in rural Georgia. She has a big garden and has always primarily eaten at home using many fresh vegetables. She does fry some foods, but I thought, after hearing about some typical meals and seeing her healthy weight, that her diet was close to her body's needs.

But what had happened to Mark? He was 12 years old with a BMI of 33 (much above the 95th percentile). He didn't play much outside. He also didn't eat his grandmother's food—he didn't like it. What did he eat? Pizza—almost every night. The pizza was a microwave version that his grandmother bought for him that he would make for himself when he got hungry. So, my question was, why was she buying the pizzas? I gave Mark's grandmother permission and support to stop buying him separate food. He could eat her food if he was hungry. The next time they came, three months later, Mark was much healthier—taller and with a slimmer appearing face. He happily showed me that his blue jeans were loose, and he announced that he was eating the vegetables his grandmother cooked and enjoyed them.

When you serve vegetables and fruit, eat them yourself and don't make a big deal out of it. Children do not respond well to pressure. Because eating is their responsibility, you should try to stay out of it as much as possible. Positive pressure ("You are doing such a good job eating your vegetables") is just as harmful as negative pressure ("You have to eat your beans"). Simply serve what you like, and then serve them again. Don't comment on how good it tastes just to get your child to eat them. But you can, of course, compliment the cook or comment on how good something is because you are really enjoying it. Remember that your role is to decide what is served and when, but your child decides if he or she eats and how much.

How to Get Your Child to Eat Broccoli

Do you like broccoli? If you don't, then you have to start by getting yourself to like it, or choose a different vegetable to serve. If you would like to try broccoli, I learned a trick that makes it taste extra good: add a teaspoon or two of lemon pepper seasoning to the water while it's cooking. You might want to toss it with a couple of teaspoons of butter after you drain off the water, or melt a slice or two of cheese over it. I like my broccoli still a little crunchy, but you might like it very soft and tender. Decide what works for you. If you really don't like broccoli, and nobody else in the family particularly likes it, forget it! There are many vegetables to try.

The proven way to get your child to eat vegetables is through consistent, positive exposure. This means that the food is on the table, and adults and other kids are eating it as one part of the meal because they enjoy it. Expect your kid to go through the following stages of interaction. It may take many times for each step.[50]

- First, they will watch you eat it.
- Then they will allow some on their plate.
- Then they will taste it—although they might spit it back out.
- Then they will swallow it.
- Finally, they will spontaneously eat some, sometimes.
- But they might change their minds at *any time*.

Kids don't go back and forth on their preferences just to drive us crazy (really!). But it will drive you crazy if you care too much whether they are eating it or not. Try your best to stop caring. Serve it in a neutral polite manner—"Would you like some peas?"—as it is passed around. Let each child say, "no, thank you," and let it be no big deal with no pressure. If he wants some, don't get excited. Just say okay and move on to the next topic of conversation. Don't watch them eat—just let them be.

Your Child Listens to You

Believe it or not, scientists have actually studied this, too. Children who are 3 to 6 years old are more likely to choose a food that they have heard an adult say was "yummy," even if the child had previously decided she didn't like it. Be assured that your child is listening to you. So if you are enjoying your vegetables, it's fine to say that you find them "really yummy."

Dinner by Candlelight

Ew. . . there are red peppers on my plate! Have you heard this at the dinner table? Now that you know you can't encourage or prompt or reward your child to eat their vegetables, what can you do? Remember that most children will eventually copy their parents, so don't worry about it if they don't take or eat any for months. Be patient, and try dinner by candlelight. My creative sister turned out the lights and served her leftover vegetable lasagna by candlelight. She had prepared it for dinner the evening before, and her 6-year-old son and 3-year-old daughter had joined forces in declaring the vegetables "yucky." So, she scooped it into containers and the next night brought out the same item reheated, but this time they had a "fancy dinner" with candles and a tablecloth. In the dim light, both kids ate more eagerly without picking out the individual pieces of peppers, spinach, and onions.

Serve Them When They Are Hungry

Another time, my sister said with a sigh that the kids didn't like the soup for dinner. Soup is one of the best (and most kid-accepted) ways to get vegetables into meals. She had made a new vegetable soup for dinner and their favorite tapioca pudding for dessert. They didn't seem to eat any of it. "Were they hungry?" I asked. Well, after she thought about it, a friend had come by not too long before dinner with some holiday cookies and other treats and they had that plus their regular snack just before that. They probably weren't hungry at all! Kids who are well-regulated will not eat again, just to eat again. So if they graze just before dinner, don't expect them to eat anything—especially unfamiliar things.

If your kids are hungry, they will eat. Kids who are not hungry don't eat—they misbehave at the table. So plan your snack and meal schedule and avoid letting your children have a snack 30 minutes before dinner.

Mix in the Vegetables

When you make the dinner, you get to choose what goes into the food. For example, soup from a can has a long list of chemicals. Soup that you put together has the extra vegetables and extra goodness that you give it—and no chemicals. Often you can make it even healthier than the original recipe calls for by adding extra vegetables. I know some parents who hide vegetables in meatloaf and burgers. It's fine to hide some vegetables, but don't always hide them. It's a balancing act. If the only way your child will eat cabbage is ground up and hidden, unseen and untasted, what will happen when she is 21 and starts to cook for herself? Will she buy and cook cabbage? Not likely. It won't look familiar.

Part of the benefit of growing up with meals that include vegetables is that you enjoy them and continue to eat them over your lifetime. So, serve recognizable vegetables and expose your child to unique flavors and textures. Not everyone will like every vegetable, and that's fine. But every child should have tasted more than just green peas.

Dr. Hansa Bhargava, a pediatrician who treats childhood obesity and has two young children age 3 years, tells me, "My twins do not like vegetables but will eat chili. So, I make chili with carrots, zucchini, spinach, onions, and tomatoes. I add a bit of ginger and a bit of canola oil (contains the good fats). They eat it, although every spoonful has to have a raisin on top. Mission accomplished!"

It's interesting that research shows that the way a food is introduced is the way it will be best accepted in the future. In one study, Drs. Sullivan and Burch introduced plain tofu, salted tofu, and sweetened tofu to three different groups of pre-schoolers.[57] Those who tried it plain wanted it that way later, and the same with the salty and sweet groups. What this means is that "doctoring" something so it will be extra appealing the first time won't necessarily help your child accept it later in a different form. Better to serve your toddler the broccoli or other new vegetables just as you would normally make these dishes and let him or her get used to the food over time.

Fruit

Fruits have lots of nutrition, and they are a delicious sweet treat—especially when they are in season. But occasionally I run into folks who have managed to overdo it. For example, one of the doctors at the hospital had decided to "be healthier," so each morning she brought to work a bag with two or three pieces of fruit sliced up as her snack. She had fruit at breakfast and lunch as well. In fact, she was getting

How to "Eat Less" Without Eating Less

A main recommendation from the American Medical Association and similar groups is for children and adults to eat fewer "energy dense" foods—foods that have a lot of calories but don't necessarily fill you up—and to increase their consumption of fruits and vegetables. You can accomplish both by mixing in the vegetables, so it's a win-win opportunity. Dr. Leahy and colleagues looked at how children reacted when they were offered pasta (macaroni and cheese or pasta with tomato sauce) with and without vegetables mixed into it.[58] They found that the children ended up eating 25% fewer calories when the pasta was mixed with vegetables, and most of the children still rated it as "yummy." Try mixing in a cup of frozen peas, corn, or green beans when you are cooking your next pasta dish.

five to six servings or more of fruit per day. One day, she quit eating all that fruit, and she noticed that she actually felt better, which really surprised her. She reported she felt less bloated. Is this possible? Well, yes. Large amounts of fruit provide large amounts of fiber and fructose. Both can increase the fuel for the bacteria in your gut and then lead to gas. Is this harmful to your child's health? No, fruit is much better than processed sweet snacks that you can buy. And has lots of vitamins and fiber and is a great healthy source of energy. A little gas is really not a big deal—but it is one of the reasons that most people will enjoy fruit in moderation. My colleague feels much better eating three servings of fruit total, instead of the four to five per day that she was getting.

Visit **www.fruitsandveggies matter.gov**, where you can plug in your child's age and gender (or your own) and find out how many cups of fruit and vegetables are recommended per day.

As his family tried to switch to fewer processed foods and get rid of the juice, John's mom bought more fruit, specifically grapes. John ate them all—at one sitting. She bought more, and he ate "the whole bowlful again." When they came back to clinic, his mom asked me if this was okay. Although it's hard to judge the health outcome completely, in general I would say that this is not enough variety. John needs about 2 cups of fruit a day. If the "whole bowl" was 3 or 4 cups, this is really too much and doesn't allow for having some fruit the rest of the day. I suggested that she offer John a snack with more foods in it, such as a piece of whole wheat toast and a glass of milk along with the grapes so he won't be so hungry and eat the whole bowlful.

Legumes—The Other Protein

Legumes are a class of vegetables that includes beans, peas, lentils, and peanuts. These are among the most versatile and nutritious foods available, but they are not well-known. In a medical school nutrition class I teach, one of my favorite "quiz" questions is to name five different legumes. Even the med students have trouble.

Legumes are plants that have pods with tidy rows of seeds inside. Peanuts are a legume that grows underground like potatoes. Sugar snap peas are usually thought of as a vegetable—but they are also part of the legume family. Soy beans are unique for their essential amino acid content, making them a great source of complete protein. They are also used to make a wide variety of foods, like tofu and soy milk, which is not so typical of the other beans in this family.

Legumes are a source of protein and low in fat. They typically contain no cholesterol, are high in folate, potassium, iron, and magnesium, and often come along with a good dose of fiber as well. Because they are a good source of protein, they can be a healthy substitute for meat.

- Most grains, fruits, and vegetables lack at least one of the essential amino acids to make complete proteins but you can combine several of these to fulfill your body's requirements for essential amino acids in the diet.
- Legumes, seeds, and whole grains should be eaten in combination and during the same day, but you don't necessarily need to eat them at the same meal.
- Here are some examples of combinations that yield complete proteins:
  - brown rice and beans
  - peanut butter and whole wheat bread
  - cornbread and pinto beans
  - refried beans with wheat or corn tortillas

Legumes come in many shapes, colors, and flavors. Limas (butter beans), fava beans (broad beans), or edamame (green soy beans) taste great in meat or vegetable stews. Black-eyed peas (cow peas) are used for fritters or bean cakes or curry dishes or mixed with ham and rice. Here in Georgia, we have many varieties of these peas at the farmer's market. Adzuki beans appear in Chinese and Japanese dishes and can also be sprouted for a crunchy salad or sandwich garnish. Lentils are common in Indian food and other eastern dishes.

Tips for Including Legumes in Your Meals

- Legumes work well in soups, stews, and casseroles. Red kidney beans go into chili or Cajun dishes, anasazi beans are used in Southwestern and Mexican side dishes and soups, and lentils are the main ingredient in the spicy Indian dish dal.
- Try chickpeas (garbanzos) or black beans (turtle beans) in salads.
- Substitute black beans for half of the meat in a recipe that calls for ground beef (or other ground meat).
- Soy nuts (roasted soy beans) can be a great snack food or salad topper.
- Serve a bean dish as the protein choice for a meal instead of meat.
- Keep a variety of canned legumes in your kitchen for a quick meal or side dish.
- If your family is new to beans, start with a small amount and increase gradually.
- Choose to have several days each week be vegetarian days; this will decrease saturated fat intake and save you money.
- Try a new legume each week. Let your child choose one and then figure out what to make with it.
- *The Moosewood Restaurant Cooks at Home* cookbook has lots of recipes that use legumes, with a focus on "fast and easy," that I have enjoyed many times (see Resources).

If you can't find a particular type of legume in the store, you can easily substitute one legume for another. For example, pinto and black beans are good substitutes for red kidney beans. And cannellini, lima beans, and navy beans are easily interchangeable. Experiment to discover which types of legumes you like best in your recipes to make your meals and snacks both nutritious and interesting.

You can buy legumes fresh, dried, canned, or frozen.

- Canned beans are fast and easy to use but can be high in sodium. To avoid this, you could buy "no added salt" products or put the beans in a colander and rinse them thoroughly before using.
- Dried beans have a fresher taste than canned beans and soaking times vary. Green peas and lentils need no soaking before cooking into soup. Soak navy beans overnight or before you leave for work before cooking into soup. Soak black beans overnight if you are putting them in the crockpot before you leave for work. *More-With-Less Cookbook* is a Mennonite cookbook and has an entire chapter on cooking with beans and lentils (see Resources).

Beating Bean Gas

Many people who eat beans have a problem with intestinal gas. Humans are missing an enzyme required to break down raffinose (a combination of three sugars) found in beans. The bacteria in our gut feast on these sugars, giving off hydrogen and carbon dioxide and causing intestinal gas. Some people avoid beans due to the intestinal gas or bloating they may produce. Starting out with small servings and gradually increasing the amount of beans you eat over several weeks can help in overcoming this. Other tips for decreasing intestinal gas from beans, peas, and lentils:

- When soaking the beans, mix ⅛ teaspoon of baking soda into the soaking water. It helps leach out the sugars, which will reduce intestinal gas.
- Drain and rinse canned beans. This will also decrease sodium.

- Don't cook beans in the water they've soaked in. The raffinose leaks into the water, and this is your chance to rinse it away.
- Change the water several times while soaking and even while cooking. This will rinse away more raffinose.

Don't Lose Your Culture

I came to this country when I was 20 years old, from Panama. A lot of things were so new to me. I had never seen pretzels or hotdogs. We had M & Ms back home, but the bags were so much bigger here. There was a lot of pressure to fit in—the kids didn't want to seem too different.

When you work, you're busy. But my family usually had a dinner on Sunday that was typical of back home—plantains, rice and beans, stewed chicken, and yucca. The other nights, it might be a sandwich or whatever you had. Gradually, we fell into the American way of eating, eating out more and not eating together. We also changed our drinking habits. For instance, Latinos drink Malta, a sweet drink, so we never drank a lot of soda in Panama. In Latin countries, we also make our own juice and nectars like papaya and tamarind. But here, our habits changed to drinking a lot of soft drinks.

When the kids went to school, they learned new foods. I had never heard of Sloppy Joes. When we moved from New York to Atlanta, we learned more new foods, like grits and biscuits. My daughter started wanting fried foods: fried chicken wings, French fries, fried everything! I knew I had to do something.

What we were losing was the habit of sitting down together to eat. In the Latin culture, we are big on family gatherings and family meals. So to find a way to do that here, I started making the dinners the day before. I gave instructions to the first person who would get home to start the rice or whatever. My son is starting to cook, and that helps a lot. One time on the bus, I sat next to a lady from Mexico. I heard her calling home and giving instructions on starting the dinner, too. That's what you have to do to make it happen.

(continued)

Don't Lose Your Culture *(Continued)*

Another challenge is that it's hard to find some of the foods from back home. I had to hunt down places that sold bacalao, the coconut, the spices. The chicken here doesn't taste like it does in Panama—it's not fresh. In Panama, you go into the market, and they kill the chicken there. When it's been shipped in a bag, it doesn't taste right, no matter what the spices.

Activity is another big difference. In Panama, the kids play outside all the time. You don't have to worry. They go to the beach to swim. We walked so much at home—to the market, to our friend's house, even to work, choir practice, and church. When I lived in New York, I walked a lot. I was so slim. If the bus didn't come, you walked. I walked from 180th to 195th and often farther. Sometimes you might not have the money for the bus fare, so you walked. Here in Atlanta, this doesn't happen. So, I have had to make an effort to walk. I walk with one of my friends in the evening, and I often ask my children to come with me. They aren't as active as they would have been in Panama, so we have to make it a priority.

—Xiomara Hinson, nutrition research assistant, Emory Children's Center

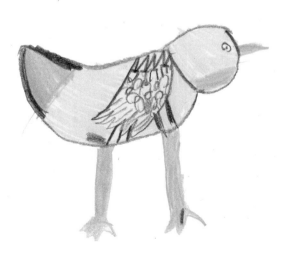

20

Wholesome Food
Is Seldom Advertised

Four young men who were part of the "lost boys," refugees from the war in Sudan, arrived in Louisville, Kentucky, one afternoon in 2001. They were assigned to an apartment that volunteers had helped arrange. That first day was bewildering for them, with new technology at every turn. Much of their young lives had been spent in a refugee camp in Kenya, after fleeing from the horrors of the war in their native Sudan. They had survived terrible hunger, sickness, and physical trials.

In the refugee camp, they ate mostly rice. They received food to eat once a day, except toward the end of the month, when, they told me, the supply would run out. Because they had been separated from their families, they lived in small groups of young men, often cousins and brothers. There were few women in the camp, and so the boys had learned to cook for themselves.

Upon their arrival in the United States, many volunteers, including my family, pitched in to get them warm clothes and to help furnish the apartment. We had been told that they might not know how to cook, so the first few days we helped them with each meal. They were unfamiliar with breakfast food like eggs and bacon or any of the cereals we put before them. At first, they politely ate what we gave them, copying what we did. But soon they got the hang of the grocery store and the can opener, and after some orientation, they figured out how to cook their own native meals in a big pot on the gas stove. They made a stew each afternoon that had onions, tomatoes, and chopped meat, often chicken. This would simmer for a few hours, and then they would make rice to serve with it. This simple four-ingredient meal is what they ate and enjoyed, day after day.

Food—and Food Products—in America

I am not sure what these four men are eating now, years later, but I hope it's something similar (with a few more vegetables). Food is cultural, part of our history and maybe our genes. In the past, most families passed their food and eating habits from generation to generation. You can see this when you travel: foods in regions of this country and in other countries are different from each other. But today, families are cooking less like their grandparents and great-grandparents.

Why? Because we are buying food "to get healthier" or because we saw an advertisement promoting that food. This change is described by Michael Pollan in his book *In Defense of Food*. Pollan points out the difference between food and food products. Food is a simple thing, produced from the earth or an animal. Food *products* are found at the grocery store *in abundance,* wrapped in layers of packaging and filled with chemicals, additives, and sweeteners that we might never otherwise eat. What these products are missing are many of the nutrients nature put into the food. These were removed so the food product can sit on grocery shelves for a long time without spoiling or growing mold. Your grandparents ate food and few, if any, food products. Did they make their own sausage or bread? My family has been dairy farmers for generations. I can still remember Aunt M's homemade yogurt, made from the fresh milk of the cows. It was creamy and rich and much better than anything I've ever had from a store.

When you buy food products, rather than food, you hand over control of the ingredients to someone else. Americans consume an estimated 140 pounds of food additives per year, of which about 110 pounds is some type of added sweetener, like corn syrup.[59] The bottom line for food manufacturers is not your health or the health of your child (no matter the message they want us to hear). The bottom line is, of course, profit, just like any other business.

Most peanut butters are food products made with sugar and emulsifiers that keep the peanut oil from separating from the peanut butter. If you buy peanut butter made with only peanuts and salt, that's a food. You'll want to mix the oil in natural peanut butter back into the peanuts before using. Keep the jar on its side or upside down to make it easier to fold in the oil.

Your Bottom Line

Your bottom line is the health of your child. Paul's mother had been worried about his weight for years, as well as her own weight. She had tried several different diets, and by the time they showed up in my office, she had found and purchased just about every low-fat product on the market. But Paul's triglycerides were still very high. I explained how triglycerides can be elevated by fructose, a simple sugar that is commonly added to foods. Paul's mother started looking for high-fructose corn syrup and sugar in the ingredients list on the food label and began to buy foods that were sweetened with an artificial sweetener instead. At the next visit, she explained that she had switched to diet breakfast cereal, diet drinks, sugar-free cookies, sugar-free chips, and more. But will this improve Paul's long-term health?

The problem with this approach is that it might not work at all. No studies have focused on whether feeding children low-sugar diet food products over the long term makes them healthier. There is evidence that sugar-substitute diet products don't really work well. I explained these studies in Chapter 12 on reducing sugar: rats fed sugar substitutes lost the ability to regulate calories, and in the Framingham studies, diet soda was associated with cardiovascular disease just like regular soda.

There are limits to what can and cannot be tested. Long-term health effects—what you really care about for your child—cannot be tested in a lab. Instead, we have all become the study subjects for those long-term effects. We can only guess what new information may come to light years from now about food products that were invented to help us avoid sugar, fat, or anything else.

The One-Change Challenge for Nutrition Research

I did a small study on children in my practice with fatty liver disease. Six families were asked to make one change: follow a "low-fructose diet" by avoiding food with fructose, high-fructose corn syrup, sugar, cane sugar, sucrose, and fruit sugar. The first discovery the parents and children made was that these ingredients are in almost every food product.

Although I designed the study to look at the effects of one change (lowering fructose), in fact, multiple changes occurred. The families ate more home-cooked meals to avoid foods with unknown ingredients. They ate more single-ingredient foods (foods without added sugar). At the end of the study, the six children had lowered their oxidative stress. Oxidative stress is an important contributor to fatty liver disease. It is the result of an imbalance between reactive oxygen products and the body's ability to absorb and disarm these reactive oxygen products. I can't state with certainty what change is responsible for this improvement . . . or if it applies to children who don't have fatty liver disease. Was the improvement because they also reduced their intake of some food additive? Did they eat more vegetables? Did they fry more . . . or less? Did they eat family-style at home, serving themselves what they wanted and stopping when they were full? The variables involved in a nutrition study are almost endless. It is very difficult to isolate one thing—like fructose—and then measure the health outcomes. This is one of the reasons why nutrition information is so confusing and sometimes contradictory.

Single-Ingredient Foods: Avoiding the Additives

Unless you're a nutrition expert, you might make yourself crazy trying to learn all the effects of each food additive (like sugar) in processed foods on long-term health. So, what do you do? Go for a simple solution: use more single-ingredient foods. Vegetables, fruits, milk, meat, whole wheat flour, black beans, pecans, almonds—these are whole foods that do not have added sugar or fat. These are foods that have been "tested" for long-term effects by generations of people. Take yourself out of the manufacturer's and advertiser's hands and regain control of what you and your family eat. Start with single-ingredient foods, like an apple, a pork chop, spinach, collard greens, onions, potatoes. (And don't be surprised if you don't see any advertising supporting this approach.)

Branding

You probably weren't aware of the first time food advertising entered into your child's life, if you are like most parents, but it starts at about age 2 years. Children's television is full of commercials. Food advertising accounts for an average of 50% of the commercials aired. If your daughter watches 3 hours of TV a day, at the end of a week, she will have

Commercials and Kids

Top First-Time In-Store Requests by Children
1. Breakfast cereal
2. Snack products
3. Beverage
4. Toy

Top Television Food Advertising Directed at Children
1. Breakfast cereal
2. Soft drinks
3. Candy
4. Salty snack products
5. Fast food

Source: Reference 47.

watched 2 full hours of food commercials.[47] Ninety percent of those commercials will be for foods high in sodium, sugars, and fats or low in nutrients.[58] If she sees an ad for simple fruits and vegetables, you can bet that it's a public service announcement.

Food manufacturers are smart. This is their chance to "brand" your child. Children quickly develop brand loyalty and preference—and it starts early. For example, if given the choice, children aged 2 and 3 years old will choose brand name products 10 to 1 over store brand products.[47] The marketers know that the first request for a specific product usually occurs around age 2 years and that 75% of the time that request occurs in a supermarket or grocery store.

Food advertising is particularly harmful for children because they don't know to question what they are seeing. They *believe* that the item will create endless fun and happiness. Four-year-old or younger children have a hard time telling the difference between the show they are watching (the entertainment) and the commercials (the pitches).

The advertisers spend a great deal of money on advertising directly to children because they know it is effective. As children's use of the Internet has increased, so has the marketing on children's Web sites. Of ten popular children's Web sites, seven had food marketing with the most advertising on www.Candystand.com.[59] Similar to TV, the foods advertised on these sites are of poor nutritional quality, including candy, sweetened breakfast cereals, fast food restaurants, chips, and the like.

Cancel Out Marketing Messages

You play an important role in shaping your child's response to advertising in general and food advertising specifically. The first step is to be aware of it. Once you start looking for food commercials, you will see that they are everywhere.

> **Top Ads on Popular Children's Web Sites**
>
> ◎ Lifesavers
> ◎ Sugar-Free Lifesavers
> ◎ Cremesavers
> ◎ McDonalds
> ◎ Cocoa Puffs
> ◎ Lucky Charms
> ◎ Trix Cereal
>
> ---
> *Source:* Adapted from Reference 61.

- ◎ Decrease your child's exposure by limiting TV time. Watch DVDs (no product advertising) or TV channels without advertising.
- ◎ Talk about commercials. Your child learns from you how to respond to media messages. By discussing the messages, you can teach your child to be skeptical of the claims and to see that the true message is "buy more."
- ◎ Don't purchase foods or visit restaurants that your child requests based on commercials. Talk about why you aren't doing this: too expensive, not necessary, not on this week's menu, or there's a similar (better?) item at home.
- ◎ Be an advocate for removing advertising from school materials and schools.

Meal Making Is Time Well-Spent

Do you know the saying "You only get out what you put in?" This is particularly true for food. We want convenient, fast food, and there are many businesses built around delivering that. However, convenient, fast food does not seem to promote lifelong health. In fact, convenient processed food has become very inconvenient as it has contributed to our obesity epidemic.

Preprepared meals are not that much more convenient. Okay, yes they do seem faster, but make sure you add in the time you used to go buy them, the extra gas, the extra expense, waiting in line, the packaging that becomes trash, and those ingredients that you would never put in your child's dinner. As a busy person, I don't cook a complicated meal every night, but I do make a nice dinner from basic ingredients every two or three nights, and then, I eat leftovers for a couple of nights. I'm delighted to have a meal waiting that just needs a little warming when I walk in the door—and I have such a sense of accomplishment. It does take a bit of planning, but I have learned to create meals from single wholesome ingredients in a very short time (see Recipes). You can, too.

The "Cost" of Processing

Let's look at oatmeal as an example. You could buy whole rolled oats, quick oats, or instant oatmeal. Oatmeal in individual packets typically has added sugar and preservatives and less fiber than the other two choices. By eating old-fashioned rolled oats or quick oats, you get more fiber and avoid the sugar. And if you want to add sugar to your cereal, you get to add just the amount you and your children like. One teaspoon of brown sugar on top is only 4 grams of sugar compared to the 13 grams in the packets.

One-Half Cup Serving	Fiber (grams)	Sugar (grams)
Whole rolled oats	4	1
Quick oats	4	1
Oatmeal packet	3	13

Tips for Finding Wholesome Food

⊚ Try a farmer's market for local, in-season fresh produce. You get wholesome food and the farmer earns a living, not the advertisers. Keeping the local farmers in business seems like a good idea (especially with transportation costs skyrocketing).

☺ Find stores that stock local produce, which tastes better. Crops that have to travel a long way to get to you are raised for storage ability and looks, not flavor. Tomatoes are a great example. The hard, waxy tomatoes that travel well do not have nearly the flavor of the soft ripe red tomatoes from the farmers market or your own backyard.

☺ Play a game with your child: While grocery shopping, see how many single-ingredient foods you can find. What about foods with two ingredients?

☺ If you do need to buy a food product, buy the one with fewer ingredients.

☺ In the grocery store, put the single-ingredient foods in the front of the cart and the multiple-ingredient ones in the back—so you can see the balance. Try to have more and more of the single-ingredient foods.

☺ Ask your grandmother or grandfather about food in their childhood. What did they eat? What were their traditions around meals?

☺ Frozen vegetables are a fast option and usually don't have many added ingredients. Keep several bags in the freezer and you can cook them up in 5 minutes. I almost always add a teaspoon of butter or a dash of olive oil after I drain them—this is only a few grams of fat but adds a lot of flavor and can make them more appealing to everyone.

☺ Canned vegetables are also a fast option, but often they have sugar or salt added. Check the labels carefully. Many vegetables have some natural sugars, so look at the ingredients list (not only the Nutrition Facts) to see what is in the can.

☺ Get other family members involved in helping create meals.

⏾ To speed things up in the evening, use a crock pot to start a meal in the morning that is ready at dinnertime.

⏾ *From Asparagus to Zucchini* is a great cookbook for ideas on how to cook fresh vegetables (see Resources).

Whole Grains

Most children and teenagers get only one serving a day of whole grains. And I am sure you have heard over and over the recommendation to eat more whole grains. I think the best reason to eat them is because they taste better! Brown rice, whole wheat flour, barley, rolled oats . . . all are whole grains. Most of them take some time to cook compared with their more processed counterparts (white rice, instant barley, and quick oats). But they have better nutrition and better flavor, along with more fiber and other micronutrients. I once brought a traditional Dutch cookie made from whole wheat flour to a potluck holiday party. One of my colleagues was delighted and explained, "When I grew up, all cookies were made with whole wheat flour, and I loved them." To her, white flour cookies "just taste bland." She said it is the same with pasta. She loves the flavor of whole wheat pasta.

Commercially produced flour varies greatly in quality, flavor, and nutritional value. Have you ever felt that a donut or bagel just sat in your stomach like a rock after you ate it? The freshness and the quality of flour used in mass production are often very low. Freshness is a major factor in the flavor and nutritional value of ground foods like flour, cornmeal, or flaxseed. I learned about this the hard way shortly after moving to Georgia. A Georgia native taught me to buy "good quality, recently dated cornmeal" in order to make good cornbread, not the stuff that had been on the shelf for who knows how long. She was right. I bought a bag of cornmeal made from corn that is grown and ground right here in Georgia and sold at a local market near my house. It made tender, moist cornbread with lots of rich corn flavor. But a month later when I reached into the pantry to get it and make cornbread again, the bag was covered in a light green mold. I had failed to read the label that suggested freezing or refrigerating it for storage. This fresh cornmeal didn't have any preservatives and had all the nutrients including the natural moisture in it, unlike the regular kind—so it spoiled more easily. I think the flavor is so good that it's worth a little bit of extra trouble to store it.

I like to bake and finding fresh whole wheat flour is another challenge. Many flours on the grocery shelves are too old to have any flavor at all. Several years ago, I read an article on flours that changed my baking completely. Some whole wheat flours are not made from grinding the whole wheat berry—they are white flour with some wheat bran mixed back in. This shocked me, but was a great explanation for why some "whole wheat" flours really don't have any more taste than white flour. I now use a traditional whole wheat flour, one that states on the package that it is made from the whole wheat berry. It should be high in both protein and fiber. My package of King Arthur Flour has 4 grams of protein and 4 grams of fiber in every ¼ cup of flour. (That food label comes in handy.) Keep your whole grains fresh and useful longer by refrigerating or freezing them, tightly sealed to keep air out.

Whole Grain "Buzz Words"

- Brown rice
- Buckwheat
- Bulgur (cracked wheat)
- Millet
- Wild rice
- Popcorn
- Quinoa
- Triticale
- Whole-grain barley
- Whole-grain corn
- Whole oats/oatmeal
- Whole rye
- Whole wheat

Source: www.cdc.gov/nccdphp/dnpa/ nutrition/nutrition_for_everyone/basics/ carbohydrates.htm#How%20much%20 carbohydrate%20do%20I%20need. Accessed October 24, 2008.

Comparing Grain—What's in ¼ Cup?		
Food	**Protein**	**Fiber**
Soft winter wheat white (White Lily)	3 grams	0 grams
Traditional whole wheat (King Arthur brand)	4 grams	4 grams
White rice, uncooked	4 grams	Less than 1 gram
Brown rice, uncooked	5 grams	3.5 grams

I have included some of my favorite recipes in the recipe section, and I have to tell you these have been a big hit with my friends and co-workers. Once you taste the rich, nutty flavor of real whole wheat, you too will have a hard time going back to a white flour cake.

Children have a preference for the familiar that helps protect them from getting into harm's way. However, when making changes to wholesome foods, that resistance can be a challenge at first. I recommend making small changes and only one at a time. Repeat the same change several times so that it has a chance to become familiar. If you have a child who resists trying new things very strongly, it is not helpful to make this a power struggle. Most children will eventually try something that they see their parents eating over and over. If you obviously don't like it, they will imitate this as well, so in that case it would be best to move on to something you do actually like.

To ease into a change, try mixing white and whole wheat flours half and half the first time you try a whole wheat recipe from this book. Use decreasing amounts of white flour each time you make the recipe.

One young mother I know recently made the switch to whole wheat pasta in her family. Her children were at the very particular ages of 4 and 6 at the time, and so she made the switch gradually to smooth the transition. She started by mixing some whole wheat pasta in with the white pasta. This helped, but of course they could see the difference in color. Over time they got used to it and then she added more until all the white pasta was gone. The whole wheat pasta has more fiber and more protein than the white flour version, making it a more wholesome choice. Now, 6 months later whole wheat is their usual, and I think the kids would be more shocked by white pasta.

Tips for Fitting Whole Grains into Meals

- Brown rice takes about an hour to cook, which can be too long for a busy night. Make twice what you need and freeze half. Reheat (microwave or steam) and serve on a busy night.
- To reheat brown rice on the stove, add a few table-spoons of water to the pan and put it over low heat for a few minutes—the steam will heat and soften the rice.
- Try different kinds of brown rice—some are more tender than others and the flavor can vary widely, just like white rice.
- Try your favorite recipe using whole wheat flour for half of the flour needed. If this works for the recipe, then try all whole wheat. Don't forget to use good quality rich, nutty whole wheat flour.

Grow Your Own

The fast food movement has also taken from us our experience of raising our own food. "It's good for everyone to be more connected with their food!" responded a friend when I said I thought it was good for children to learn more about growing food. She pointed out the bigger truth. We have all become too distant from the sources of our food, and it hurts us in many ways—we don't get the quality that we would want, we don't put the effort into acquiring the food, and we value it less—therefore wasting it and losing money.

My parents gardened all through my childhood, and now all five of us "kids" have gardens, too—even my brother who

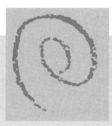

Question for the Psychologist

Q **My son wants me to give him money for eating healthier, just like his friend's mother does. This seems like a bad idea to me. Can it be good to reward him for what he should be doing anyway?**

A This is an excellent question. If you reward kids for what they naturally like to do, you run the risk of interfering with the natural pleasure and intrinsic rewards they get from doing what is good and right. You don't want them to grow up always expecting and demanding a reward. I suggest a temporary use of rewards to help shape the behaviors of our children when needed. If your son is strongly resisting the changes to healthier eating, you might give him rewards for a while, for example a reward for cooperating for 1 week with the food plan. Don't "pay" him, but offer instead activities such as watching a movie together, extra playtime with a favorite toy, staying up an extra half hour, playing a board game with you, having a friend over, and so on. If your child is little, you may need to give a reward immediately after the cooperation, and these rewards need to be smaller: a sticker, an extra story that night, sitting in your lap for a while right after dinner. I predict that once your child has become used to the new habits, he won't need these rewards anymore. Then you tell him that he no longer needs special rewards for cooperating with the food plan, and that you are proud of how grown up he has become.

lives in an apartment with his wife and baby in New York City. They joined a cooperative garden in a formerly vacant lot just around the corner from their home and grow tomatoes, herbs, and even strawberries. My older sister Jolene has a small garden in the back of her yard (with a carefully constructed rabbit fence), and both of her kids love to help. My sister Margaret's husband Ben is the gardener in her family—and Adam, her 4-year-old son, is a champion vegetable picker. My sister Sarah and her husband have a shady backyard but still manage to have a big patch of tomatoes and herbs along the garage with lots of help from their three sons.

Jolene grows cherry tomatoes, among other things, and last summer she had a small bowl of the ripe fruits on the kitchen table. One of her college students had come over to babysit, and as Jolene was getting ready to leave, the young lady picked up a tomato and commented, "I know I should eat this because it's good for me—so I will eat it—but I am going to swallow it whole so I don't have to taste it."

My sister was shocked—and suggested the student not eat it. Those cherry tomatoes were the product of almost 3 months of work, and in the cool summers of Michigan, the plants don't produce very long. Jolene, her husband, and kids all loved the sweet, tangy, bright red fruits . . . and Jolene wasn't ready to have someone eat one just because she "ought to," not to mention without chewing it! Knowing our food changes our relationship to it. Jolene was attached to her cherry tomatoes; she valued them, but her babysitter did not.

You can grow something to eat, and your children will benefit from the experience. An easy way to start is to grow some herbs in a pot. Rosemary is delicious on meats and roasted potatoes. In the spring and summer, basil grows in a pot pretty easily. Most local hardware and garden stores have a whole selection of herbs in the spring. You can plant a large pot with several different herbs and place it in a sunny spot outside. If you don't have any outdoor space, try a small rectangular planter in a sunny window. Fresh herbs are great in salads, soups, and main dishes and for roasting almost anything.

Chicken Little and "the Girls"

I have chickens—three to be exact. I am sure you are thinking what most people do . . . chickens?! I live in the city, in the middle of Atlanta, in a neighborhood called Decatur. Decatur was a little town before Atlanta got so big, so it has a nice small town feeling and a center square and our own city ordinances allowing chickens. Two of my neighbors also have chickens.

And there is a "how to raise chickens in the city" class each fall and spring at our local community garden.

I first wanted chickens because of my friend Martha, who lives on 5 acres in Kentucky. After she and her husband bought their place, they built a small barn and made the back end into a chicken coop. She has a nice big fenced pasture for her dozen chickens to range on during the day. I love visiting her place and seeing the chickens, and the fresh eggs tasted amazing—so much flavor and bright yellow yolks. When I moved to Atlanta, I looked into the ordinances and like many cities, chickens are allowed. My three hens (girl chickens) don't make much noise—except the occasional proud "boooock-bock-bock" when someone lays an egg. They sleep in a small house, a little larger than a big doghouse in the corner of my yard. In the morning, I let them out to wander the yard and at dusk they tuck themselves back into the henhouse. I just close the door for safe keeping so the raccoons or possums won't get them. Chickens don't fly much (depends on the breed), and so mine mostly stay in the yard. Once one flew over the fence while I was at work, but she was rescued by Hannah, a little girl down the street. She knew about chickens, and so she just chased it back up my driveway.

I have chickens because I like being part of the food cycle. I have food scraps, which the chickens eat. They love to eat leftovers. They also love to eat cheese, bread, and lettuce, and although they aren't really "pets," they do come running to see if I have food for them when I go into the yard. One of them is a little smaller, so I named her "Chicken Little." The other two are just "the girls." I like having an organic garden, and the chickens really reduce the insect population. They eat insects, especially the big "palmetto bugs" that abound in our woodsy neighborhood (known as cockroaches just about everywhere else), weeds, and weed seeds. They peck around the yard digging up the dirt while hunting for bugs and loosen the soil. They "compost" and "fertilize" by spreading little bits of chicken poop around the yard—although with only three and a medium-sized yard, it's not that noticeable. They do eat some of my flowers, and they love ripe cherry tomatoes. I have to use temporary chicken wire structures to protect certain plants at certain times. But I have to say, watching a chicken leap 4 feet up in the air to pluck a ripe cherry tomato off the plant is almost better than eating the tomato! I will definitely be growing cherry tomatoes again next year, for all of us.

They lay delicious eggs for me to collect each day. I get one to two eggs per day. Often as I arrive home from work, my neighbor Harper Rae (now 4 years old) will call through the fence to see if she can come over and "see the chickens." She and her mom and sometimes her older brother Hogan will come over, bringing along their leftover vegetable scraps for the chickens to eat. Rae also knows that the chickens love corn on the cob (their favorite), apple cores, and leftover lettuce. I love watching Rae and Hogan check the nests for eggs and their excitement when they find two! They are learning the cycle of food—and the value of each egg. If one gets dropped, we have to wait until tomorrow to find new ones and only if the "girls" lay some that day.

Because of this, I am very connected to the eggs I eat. When I crack one open for breakfast, I know a lot about what went into making that egg. On a deeper level, I think it is important to understand how food is made and where it comes from. It does not start wrapped in plastic with sugar and flavoring added. The preservatives were not in there when it grew from the ground. Sometimes, I have leftover food from a restaurant, and I stop to think whether it's healthy enough for my chickens . . . and I ate it? I shouldn't be putting anything in my body that I have concerns about. My chickens remind me on a daily basis about how I'm connected to our food chain.

Getting in Touch with Your Food

Not everyone can raise chickens. In fact, I don't think I have convinced even one person to get chickens yet (although I keep trying). But everyone can get closer to their food sources by going to the farmer's market and meeting the people who grow and raise the food, by growing something in your own yard or in a pot on your deck or windowsill, and by participating in community supported agriculture (CSA).

In a book on farm produce, John Hendrickson points out that since 1900, 97% of fruit and vegetable varieties have become unavailable commercially. How does this change affect us? At grocery stores we can always find Red Delicious and Granny Smith apples. How about a Jersey Mac, Paula Red, or Northern Spy apple? Wouldn't you like to taste one of these? Unfortunately, they don't keep well in storage, so you can only find them at local orchards and markets after the harvest in the fall. When we handed over the choice of what will be grown to food manufacturers, we lost a lot. Keeping local farmers in business—and encouraging them to grow a wide variety of vegetables and fruits—is good for our health, too.

Many of my friends have joined a CSA. A CSA is composed of three groups: the farmers, a core group of organizers, and the consumers. By joining and becoming one of the consumers, you receive a share of the produce from the farmers each week. Typically this is a basketful of in-season vegetables. Some CSAs send recipe suggestions for the vegetables as well, and many encourage you and your children to visit and see where the food comes from. Some CSAs invite members to help harvest the crops. This is a great way to connect with your food.

For help finding a CSA near you, go to **www.biodynamics.com/csa** or **www.localharvest.org.**

My sister Jolene's daughter loves strawberries, so they go strawberry picking as a family. Instead of buying the big but low-flavor strawberries they have in the grocery store most of the year, they have a freezer full of individual bags of locally grown, full-of-flavor strawberries. Some years they don't pick enough to last, so they get frozen supermarket ones . . . and even Alice, who is just 5 years old, notices the decrease in flavor.

Parent Tips on Making a Healthy Kitchen

- ◎ We buy lots of foods in bulk—saves money and there is no advertising on them.
- ◎ We prepare the evening meal together as a family and then sit down to enjoy it. This gives us a chance to reconnect with one another and unwind from the day. Cooking together shows our daughter how food is prepared and how to cooperate and clean up and gives her quality time with mommy and daddy. She really looks forward to this "kitchen time."
- ◎ If you don't buy junk food, it's not in your kitchen to be eaten. Stock up on healthy snacks and foods.
- ◎ The family farmer is more important than the family doctor. We believe that "you are what you eat." This includes where your food comes from and how it is raised. Good, clean, fair, organic food is preventative medicine.
- ◎ We use cookbooks as inspiration for trying out new foods or preparing familiar foods in new ways. The first time I use a new recipe, I follow the directions. Later on, I may use that recipe as a starting point for creating my own dish. We think recipes should be guides, not rules; be creative. If you have good ingredients and mix them with care, you usually get a delicious (though seldom repeatable) meal. But that's okay—that meal will be one of a kind, and remind us how special it is to be able to eat and enjoy.

—Michelle and Joel Kimmons, PhD
CDC Nutrition, Physical Activity and Obesity Division

Benefits of Local Food

Buying from your local farmer's market is a great way to find fresh local food that is not processed. Vegetables that are in season are usually more flavorful. Sometimes you can find local meats and cheeses that have fewer additives than grocery store meats. You also are benefiting the world that your children live in—by choosing foods that haven't traveled as far and foods that are not wrapped in layers of packaging made from precious resources and heading to the garbage dump. Choosing local fresh food benefits your child and your child's world.

Benefits of Organic Food

There are several reasons why organic food may be healthier for you and your child compared with foods that are conventionally grown with pesticides or additives like growth hormones. It won't surprise you if I point out that organic foods often taste better—and that is a great benefit as well. Multiple studies have shown that organically and sustainably grown vegetables, including tomatoes, strawberries, corn, blueberries, and more contain more antioxidants than conventionally grown vegetables.[62-64] A recent study demonstrated that organic milk has two times the antioxidants compared with nonorganic and it has a better ratio of good fats to "bad" fats.[65] Foods that are conventionally grown also may have pesticides still on them. For foods that you peel, like oranges and avocados, this may be less important than for foods that have lots of crevices and creases like green peppers, lettuce, kale, and strawberries.

Because organic farmers have more expenses and are not typically government subsidized, organic food is often more expensive. So, it's usually necessary to make choices. For me, I pick and choose what I buy organic. I like to buy organic vegetables that are in season, especially at the farmer's market. I only buy organic dairy products (milk, butter, cheese) because I know that the organic version tastes better and has more antioxidants. Organic dairy also has fewer antibiotics and growth hormones than regular dairy.

In our food supply system, you "vote" with your dollars by buying the foods you think are the healthiest for your family. This keeps organic and local farmers in business. You can also let your community and political leaders know that you want access to plentiful, varied, fresh, local vegetables and not just "the big three" foods (corn, soybeans, and wheat) that are heavily subsidized by our tax dollars.

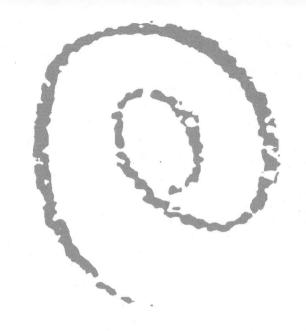

Recipes and
Snack Suggestions

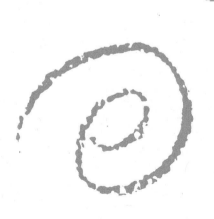

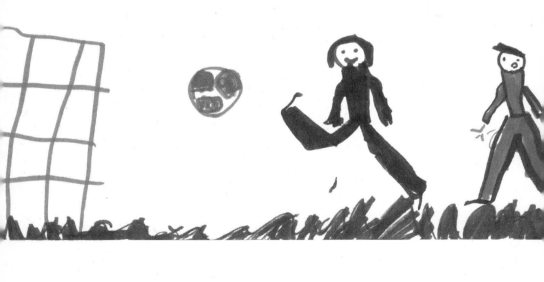

Healthy, Delicious Home-Cooked Foods

*I*f you plan ahead, you can make and serve meals made from single, wholesome ingredients in a very short time. In the pages ahead, I've shared my personal favorite and family recipes. I also asked professional chefs and dietitians to contribute their kid-friendliest dishes. I hope you find guidance and support in the recipes and food ideas that follow. As you try the recipes, feel free to adapt them to include ingredients that are your favorites.

Ways to Serve More Whole Grains

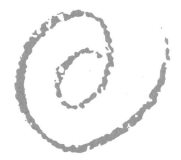

Use fresh, high-quality whole grains. Buy traditional whole wheat flour, which is made from the whole wheat berry. Fresh stone-ground corn meal makes the moistest cornbread. These grains do not last more than a week on the shelf, so store them in air-tight containers in the refrigerator. You can also freeze them in 1-cup portions with the air removed.

Fireside Oatmeal

Jennifer DeLuca

½   cup rolled oats (old fashioned)
¼   cup seedless raisins
¼   tsp. ground cinnamon
⅛   tsp. allspice

1   tsp. granulated sugar
1½   tsp. molasses
¾   cup water

Combine oats, raisins, cinnamon, allspice, and sugar in a microwave-safe cereal bowl. Add molasses and water to bowl and stir. Place uncovered bowl in microwave and cook on high for 90 seconds. Remove bowl from microwave and stir. Let oatmeal sit for 1 minute before serving.

Makes 2 servings.

Easy Oatmeal Pancakes

Miriam Vos

I can put this batter together while my cast-iron pan is heating up—takes about 5 minutes. The waffles have a rich, nutty flavor from the oatmeal and the whole wheat flour and are so moist that I often don't even bother with putting syrup on them.

½   cup rolled oats (old fashioned)
1   dash salt
1   egg, beaten
½   cup whole wheat flour

1   cup water
2   tsp. butter
⅛   cup milk
1   tsp. baking powder

Combine oats, water, and salt in a large microwave-safe bowl. Cook uncovered on high for 1 minute. Remove from microwave and stir. Return to microwave and cook on high for 30 seconds. Stir in butter and set on counter to "rest" for 1 minute. Add egg and milk to oatmeal mixture. Add flour and baking powder. Mix all ingredients together for 10 seconds. Cook pancakes in a preheated cast-iron pan.

Makes 12 pancakes.

Whole Wheat Cinnamon French Toast with Applesauce Vanilla Topping

Ellen Stokes

4	eggs	1	cup 2% milk
10–12	slices whole wheat	1	Tbsp. butter
	cinnamon raisin bread	1	cup unsweetened applesauce
2–3	drops vanilla extract		

Whisk eggs and milk together in a shallow bowl. Soak bread slices in mixture, flipping slices until liquid is absorbed. Cook on griddle or in frying pan in small amounts of butter until browned on both sides. For topping, combine applesauce and vanilla and heat on stove in a small pan. Top with warm applesauce topping and serve immediately.

Extra slices of cooked French toast can be wrapped individually and frozen. Reheat in toaster oven.

Banana-Buckwheat Pancakes

Charles Loomis

These are a tasty treat. You can hardly tell the difference between these buckwheat pancakes and the traditional white flour style.

¾	cup buckwheat flour	¾	cup whole wheat flour
½	tsp. baking soda	1	tsp. sea salt
1	cup buttermilk	¾	cup milk
1	Tbsp. honey	1	tsp. cinnamon
2	large eggs	2	Tbsp. safflower oil
3	large, ripe bananas,		Cinnamon
	sliced into 1-inch slices		Maple syrup

Mix the dry ingredients together in one bowl. Mix the wet ingredients together in separate bowl. Combine both mixtures, just barely incorporating them together. Add the bananas and gently stir them in, about 5 stirs with a wooden spoon. Heat a nonstick skillet or pan over medium heat. Lightly grease the pan with a little bit of oil. Ladle the mix into the pan ¼ cup at a time. When the top of the pancake starts to bubble, check the bottom for doneness. When it is golden brown, it is time to flip. Cook the second side until it is also golden brown. Sprinkle with cinnamon and serve with maple syrup.

Whole-Grain Waffles

Miriam Vos

1¾ cups traditional whole wheat flour (King Arthur brand preferred)	½ cup rolled oats (old fashioned, chopped in blender several times to make smaller) or quick-cooking oats
½ tsp. baking soda	
1½ tsp. baking powder	
1 tsp. sugar	½ tsp. salt
2 eggs	1¾ cups buttermilk (or 1¼ cups plain yogurt combined with ½ cup milk)
6 Tbsp. melted butter	

In a large bowl, combine all dry ingredients. In a separate bowl, whisk eggs, then add buttermilk and butter. Combine dry and wet mixtures with a few broad strokes, just until combined. Cook on preheated waffle iron that has been sprayed with nonstick cooking spray. Waffles will keep for a week and heat up easily in the toaster.

Makes 12 waffles.

Whole Wheat Biscuits

Miriam Vos

I like to add a few tablespoons of oat bran or flax seeds to make hearty breakfast biscuits.

1¾ cup traditional whole wheat flour (King Arthur brand preferred)	¼ tsp. salt
½ tsp. baking soda	2 tsp. baking powder
¾ cup buttermilk (or ½ cup plain yogurt, thinned with ¼ cup milk)	5 Tbsp. butter, chilled

Preheat oven to 425°F. Combine dry ingredients in a large bowl. Cut in butter with pastry blender. Add buttermilk and mix lightly. Turn dough out onto floured board and pat or roll to 1-inch thickness. Use a biscuit cutter to cut out the biscuits from flattened dough. Bake on a greased cookie sheet for 10–12 minutes, until biscuits are lightly browned.

The sourness of the buttermilk or yogurt make these extra tender, but if you need to use plain milk, use slightly less than ¾ cup. For less fuss and clean up, instead of rolling out the dough, just scoop spoonfuls onto the cookie sheet. For crispy biscuits, bake far apart. For softer biscuits, bake close together. The best flavor is obtained from using the best whole wheat flour.

Makes 12 biscuits.

Sweet Potato & Blueberry Pancakes

Chef David Bressler

For a quicker preparation, microwave the sweet potatoes until tender or prepare them a day or night before or make several batches and freeze in 1¼-cup portions.

1½	cup whole wheat flour	1½	cups milk
1¼	cups sweet potatoes	1–2	cups fresh or frozen blueberries
¼	cup butter, melted	2	large eggs, beaten
1	additional Tbsp. butter or canola oil for frying	3	tsp. baking powder
½	tsp. ground nutmeg	1	tsp. salt

Peel and quarter sweet potatoes. Add potatoes to a pot of boiling water. Boil until soft. Mash potatoes and allow to cool to room temperature before making batter.

In a large mixing bowl, sift together flour, baking powder, salt, and nutmeg. In a separate bowl, combine milk, potatoes, eggs, and butter. Combine the two mixtures until dry ingredients are just moistened. Allow batter to set for about 15 minutes.

Heat a griddle or skillet to medium-high heat. Lightly grease griddle with butter. Drop batter by heaping tablespoons onto griddle or skillet. Add blueberries and fry, turning once, until golden brown on both sides. Serve with real maple syrup or without a topping if the blueberries are fresh and sweet already.

Breakfast Muffins

Miriam Vos

1	cup water	1	cup raisins
1¼	cup traditional whole wheat flour	1	cup rolled oats
1½	cup wheat bran	1½	tsp. baking soda
1	cup buttermilk		

Preheat oven to 350°F. Simmer raisins and water for 5 minutes and set aside to cool slightly. In large bowl, stir together dry ingredients. In a separate bowl, combine simmered water and raisins and buttermilk. Stir the liquid ingredients into the dry ingredients, just barely combining. Scoop mixture into greased muffin tins or into a loaf pan. Bake muffins for 20 minutes; bake loaf for 1 hour or until toothpick comes out clean.

Makes 12 muffins or 1 loaf.

Pumpkin-Carrot Muffins

Jill Nussinow, MS, RD (The Veggie Queen)

1 large egg	2 Tbsp. canola oil
½ cup mashed cooked or canned pumpkin	1 large carrot, grated
1 tsp. vanilla extract	1 cup milk or soymilk
⅔ cup sugar	2 cups whole wheat flour
1 Tbsp. baking powder	½ tsp. salt
¼ cup currants or raisins	1 tsp. cinnamon
Nonstick cooking spray	⅓ cup chopped walnuts

Preheat oven to 375°F. Spray 12-muffin tin with cooking spray. In a medium bowl, beat egg. Add the oil, pumpkin, carrots, vanilla, and soymilk. Stir well to combine. In a separate large bowl, thoroughly combine flour, sugar, salt, baking powder, and cinnamon. Stir in currants and walnuts. Fold the wet ingredients into the dry ingredients until just combined. Spoon the batter into the muffin tins until each is ⅔ full.

Bake for 20–25 minutes until a toothpick or other tester comes out clean. Remove from oven. Let cool in the tin for 5 minutes, then remove from tin and place on baking rack to cool.

Makes 12 muffins.

Super Moist Corn Muffins

Miriam Vos

For extra spicy muffins, add 1–2 Tbsp. of chopped, drained chilis.

1 cup whole wheat flour	1 cup white or yellow cornmeal, stone ground if possible
½ tsp. salt	
2 tsp. sugar	2 tsp. baking powder
½ tsp. baking soda	1 large egg, lightly beaten
3 Tbsp. butter, melted, cooled slightly	1 cup plain yogurt
½ cup milk	1 cup corn kernels, canned (drained) or frozen (thawed)

Grease and flour 12 muffin cups or line with paper liners. Heat oven to 375°F. In a mixing bowl, combine the cornmeal, flour, salt, baking powder, soda, and sugar. In a small bowl, stir together the egg, yogurt, milk, and melted butter; stir into the flour mixture just until blended. Stir in corn. Fill prepared muffin cups about ¾ full. Bake for 20–25 minutes, or until lightly browned.

Makes 12 muffins.

Cranberry Cake

Jolene Vos

2¼	cups frozen or fresh cranberries	2	eggs, beaten
1	tsp. vanilla	¾	cup sugar
1	cup whole wheat flour	¾	cup butter, melted

If using frozen berries, let thaw before beginning. Preheat oven to 375°F. Spread the cranberries on the bottom of a 9-inch pie pan and set aside. In a medium mixing bowl, beat eggs with a whisk then stir in vanilla and sugar. Mix well. Add flour and mix. Add melted butter. Pour or spread batter over cranberries. Bake for 40 minutes.

Makes 8 servings.

Carrot Cake

Miriam Vos

1	cup whole wheat flour (King Arthur preferred)	1	cup all-purpose white flour
1⅓	cup sugar	2	tsp. baking soda
1	cup canola oil or 2 sticks butter, melted	3	eggs, lightly beaten
2	tsp. vanilla extract	1¼	cup finely shredded raw carrots, packed
1	cup coconut	1	cup walnuts (optional)
1	can cream cheese frosting	¾	cup drained, crushed pineapple, in juice not syrup

Preheat the oven to 350°F. Grease a 13 × 9–inch baking dish. Stir together the flour, sugar, and soda. Add the oil, eggs, and vanilla and beat well. Fold in carrots, walnuts, coconut, and pineapple. Pour batter into pan and bake until toothpick comes out clean (about 1 hour). Cool and frost or serve without frosting.

Easy Whole Wheat Pie Crust

Miriam Vos

1¼	cups traditional whole wheat flour	1	tsp. sugar
¼	tsp. salt	7	Tbsp. chilled unsalted butter
3	Tbsp. ice water (approximate)		

Combine flour, sugar, and salt. Add butter and cut into small pea-size pieces and the mixture resembles coarse meal. This can be done in a food processor using on/off turns. Sprinkle ice water over mixture while stirring and blend until moist clumps form. Gather mixture into a ball and wrap in plastic. Chill for 1 hour (or longer) and then roll out to desired size.

Makes 1 crust for 10-inch pie pan.

Rustic Whole Wheat Fruit Tart

Miriam Vos

4	apples or pears, cored, or 5–6 plums, pitted	1	whole wheat pie crust, unbaked
1	tsp. butter, in pieces	1	tsp. sugar

Slice fruit into ½-inch thick slices in a pie pan to contain the juice. Roll out crust and place in a 10-inch pie pan or on a cookie sheet. Layer fruit in concentric circles, leaving 2 inches of dough at the outside clear of fruit. Fold up the edges of the dough toward the center all the way around. Sprinkle the top of the fruit with sugar and dot with butter.

Bake at 400°F for 10 minutes and then turn down to 350°F and bake until the fruit is tender to touch using a fork (about 45 minutes). Let cool for at least 10–15 minutes and serve.

Makes 6 servings.

Whole Wheat Brownies

Jolene Vos

½	cup butter	2	oz. unsweetened chocolate
1	cup sugar	¾	cup whole wheat flour
1	tsp. baking powder	1	tsp. vanilla
2	eggs, beaten		

Preheat over to 350°F. Melt the butter and chocolate in a small saucepan over low heat. In a separate bowl, mix together the sugar, flour, and baking powder. Combine the flour mixture with the butter and chocolate. Add vanilla and eggs. Pour batter into an 8-inch buttered cake pan. Bake for 30 minutes. Let cool and slice.

Makes 9 servings.

Whole Wheat Oatmeal Cookies

Miriam Vos

I prefer to make them smaller in size and offer several in a serving. Great with a glass of milk.

2	sticks butter (1 cup), at room temperature	1¼–1½	cup dark brown sugar
		1	tsp. milk powder
2	eggs	2	tsp. vanilla
1½	cup whole wheat flour (King Arthur preferred)	1	tsp. baking soda
		2	Tbsp. flax seeds
½	cup sunflower seeds	3	cup rolled oats
¼	tsp. salt (use more if using unsalted butter)	1	cup raisins or real chocolate chips or mixture

Preheat oven to 350°F. In large bowl, mix butter, brown sugar, and milk powder until creamy. Blend in eggs and vanilla until light and fluffy. Add flour and baking soda; mix. Stir in remaining ingredients. Scoop by tablespoonfuls onto lightly greased cookie sheets. Bake for 10 minutes or until lightly browned.

Makes 60 small cookies.

Focus on Vegetables

It's worth buying fresh vegetables from the farms around where you live. Fresh vegetables are full of nutrients and taste. You can freeze fresh vegetables if you have a deep freezer or buy frozen vegetables when things are out of season. Most stores will have better prices when a particular vegetable is in season. For example, avocados are cheaper in early spring. Cantaloupes are cheaper in the summer. Tomatoes are tastiest in late summer and fall. If you shop at a farmer's market, grow your own, or belong to a community-supported agriculture group, you will also learn when things are in season and you can get some of the freshest, best-tasting vegetables. Vegetables that are bred to travel long distances are not nearly as tasty as locally grown ones. *Simply in Season* and *From Asparagus to Zucchini* are both great cookbooks that give recipes by season, helping you to focus on vegetables and to use what is fresh now (see Resources).

For cooking, I primarily use olive oil and canola oil. Both extra virgin and virgin olive oils are cold-pressed olives, a process that retains the olive nutrients. "Virgin" on the label also means the makers haven't cut the product with chemically processed oils. An open bottle of olive oil will last for up to 3 months if you keep it in a cool, dry, dark pantry or cabinet. Olive oil doesn't tolerate high-heat frying but works fine for low-to-medium–heat cooking. Canola oil is multipurpose, with a mild flavor.

Sweet Potato Fries

Miriam Vos and Michelle McKenzie

These can be made with almost any version of potato—yams, sweet potato, the white sweet potato you find in Puerto Rico, or even white potatoes. Leaving the peel adds extra fiber.

    2   large sweet potatoes with skins on
  1–2 Tbsp. olive oil
      Salt to taste
      Fresh rosemary, finely chopped, and/or chili powder (optional)

Preheat oven to 400°F. Scrub and clean potatoes, cutting out any bad spots. Cut potatoes in half. Place each half face down onto a cutting board and cut into slices lengthwise. Turn each slice onto its side and cut into strips, almost square. Put the strips onto a baking sheet and drizzle with olive oil. Hand toss to coat all sides. Sprinkle salt and seasonings lightly over fries to taste. Bake until tender, usually 15 to 30 minutes depending on size and type of potato strips, turning once. Cooked potatoes can stand at room temperature for up to 3 hours or can be refrigerated for up to 3 days; recrisp leftovers in a 450°F oven for several minutes.

Makes 6 servings.

Crispy Grilled Eggplant

Miriam Vos

    2   medium eggplants
  1–2 Tbsp. olive oil
      Salt to taste

Preheat grill to medium. Wash and dry eggplants. Slice eggplants into ½-inch circles. Using fingers or a brush, lightly rub both sides of each slice with olive oil. Place on grill. Turn when browned on one side. Cook until center is tender. Salt to taste and serve.

Makes 6 servings.

Grilled Okra

Miriam Vos

You will need a vegetable grilling basket for this. This is the only "unslimy" okra you will ever eat—even okra haters often like it! This recipe can be used for many vegetables and combinations of vegetables. Some other favorites are red peppers, onions, squash, and mushrooms. Just chop them up into 1-inch pieces, toss them with olive oil and salt, and throw them into the basket.

1	lb. okra		1	Tbsp. olive oil
⅛	tsp. salt			

Heat grill. Wash okra and cut off stems. Toss okra with olive oil and a pinch of salt. Put into a vegetable basket designed for grills. Cook over medium heat. Turn and toss every 2–3 minutes, more often if the grill is very hot. When done, okra should look dry and slightly wilted, but not blackened.

Makes 6 servings.

Roasted Root Vegetables

Miriam Vos

1	large white potato		1	medium sweet potato
3–4	carrots		1	small winter squash
1–2	tsp. olive oil			(butternut is one of the easier
½	tsp. salt			ones to peel)
1	tsp. fresh or dried rosemary, thyme, or oregano			

Preheat oven to 350°F. Scrub skins of potatoes and carrots. Cut out any bad spots; peel only if necessary. Chop into 1-inch pieces. Put in 9 × 13 inch or larger baking dish. Cut squash in half and scoop out the seeds. Place the squash face down and cut again into quarters or smaller pieces that you can easily hold in your hand. Carefully remove skin with peeler or sharp knife. Put squash pieces in pan with other vegetables. Drizzle with olive oil. Sprinkle with salt and herbs. Using your hands, mix vegetables to coat all sides with oil, salt, and herbs. Place in oven. Bake until tender, about 1 hour, stirring once or twice to avoid scorching.

Makes 6 servings.

Blushing Mashed Potatoes

Ellen Stokes

Yukon Gold potatoes have a naturally buttery taste, so you don't need much butter. To save for later meals, freeze potatoes in individual portions on a cookie sheet lined with waxed paper. Once portions are frozen solid, put in plastic bags. Reheat in microwave.

3½	lb. gold potatoes	¾	lb. carrots
1	cup 2% milk, warmed	1	Tbsp. butter
	Garlic powder, salt, pepper to taste		

Peel potatoes (if desired) and cut into 2-inch pieces. Scrub carrots and cut into 1-inch pieces. Boil potatoes and carrots in separate saucepans until tender. Drain and mash separately with hand masher or mixer. Combine milk and butter in a saucepan and heat until butter melts. Pour milk mixture into potatoes and whip by hand. Add mashed carrots. Season to taste with garlic powder, salt, and pepper. Serve immediately.

Makes 6–8 servings.

Eggplant Parmesan

Xiomara Hinson

Kids love to grate their own cheese. Look for a nice hard-cheese grater at a kitchen store. When I don't have much time for dinner, I will often cook some whole wheat pasta, sprinkle it with olive oil, and serve with fresh grated parmesan cheese. This, along with some frozen vegetables cooked in 5 minutes, is a super-fast healthy dinner as well.

1	eggplant	½	cup spaghetti sauce (look for
½	cup fresh grated parmesan cheese		one with little added sugar)
2	Tbsp. olive oil	1	tsp. oregano

Wash eggplant and cut into 1-inch-thick circles. Use fingers or brush to coat with oil. Cook in skillet or on grill over medium-high heat until eggplant is brown on both sides. Place browned eggplant in baking dish. Pour spaghetti sauce over eggplant and sprinkle with grated parmesan cheese. Bake or grill for 15 minutes until warm and cheese is melted. Alternatively, cook in microwave on high for 6 minutes.

Make 4 servings.

Mashed Cauliflower

Xiomara Hinson

This will taste a little more like mashed potatoes if you add 2 medium white or gold potatoes, which are a little drier and have a creamier texture than cauliflower. Wash and cube the potatoes and cook and mash them with the cauliflower.

1 head cauliflower	½ cup plain yogurt
1 Tbsp. butter	(more or less to taste)
Salt and pepper to taste	

Wash cauliflower and remove leaves. In a large saucepan with cover, steam or simmer whole head in small amount of water until tender. Drain well. Mash in pan with potato masher or mixer until cauliflower is smooth. Stir in yogurt, butter, and salt and pepper to taste.

Basic Braised Greens

Michelle McKenzie

⅓ cup olive oil	4 garlic cloves, finely chopped
Pinch red pepper	or mashed
1 tsp. honey (optional)	2 cups chicken or vegetable stock
3 lb. kale or other winter	Splash Sherry or apple cider
braising greens (mustard or	vinegar
collard greens), stems diced and	Extra virgin olive oil for serving
leaves coarsely chopped	1 Tbsp. pine nuts, toasted, for
Salt and freshly ground pepper	topping (optional)

Heat oil in a wide pot over medium heat. Add the garlic and red pepper flakes; cook over moderately high heat, stirring, just until fragrant, about 30 seconds. Add the stock and bring to a boil. Add the kale in large handfuls, letting it wilt slightly before adding more. Season with salt and pepper, then cover and cook over moderate heat until the kale is all wilted, about 5 minutes. Reduce the heat to medium-low, remove the lid and cook until the liquid has evaporated, about 25 minutes. To serve, drain, transfer to a bowl, drizzle with fresh olive oil, and top with pine nuts, if desired.

Makes about 6 servings.

Suggestions for leftover greens:

- Make a unique pesto topping for hot pasta by combining greens in a food processor with a handful of toasted pine nuts, garlic cloves (to taste), drizzle of olive oil, and a squeeze of lemon. Pulse until finely ground.
- Add at the end of cooking to a hot winter soup or stew. Especially good in bean soup.
- Substitute for the usual spinach in lasagna.
- Adds texture to a vegetable frittata (see recipe, page 237).

Vegetable Frittata

Michelle McKenzie

Experiment by adding different leftover vegetables or a fabulous local cheese, like asparagus with fresh chevre or boiled and chopped potatoes with cheddar. Leftovers can be sandwiched between bread with a little mayo, sliced onion, and tomato for healthy and delicious weekday lunch.

1 cup or so leftover braising greens or other vegetable, chopped and cooked	1 Tbsp. extra virgin olive oil
6 eggs	1 Tbsp. unsalted butter
3 Tbsp. fresh or dried parsley, chopped	½ cup pecorino or other type of romano cheese, finely grated
	Salt and pepper to taste

Preheat oven broiler. In a bowl, whisk eggs until frothy. Stir in remaining ingredients. Heat a medium sauté pan over medium-high heat and melt the butter. Add the egg mixture and cook until the bottom begins to set, about 7–10 minutes. Place the pan under the preheated broiler and continue cooking until the eggs are completely set and cooked through and the top is lightly browned, about 3–5 minutes.

Gently shake the pan to loosen the frittata and slide it onto a serving plate. Cut into wedges and serve warm or at room temperature.

Roasted "Pumpkin" and Red Quinoa Pilaf

Michelle McKenzie

This interesting pilaf is a great side to meat or fish and a tasty lunch box addition when sent to school in a soup thermos. Kids tend to love anything with "pumpkin," and the deep crimson color of the red quinoa intrigues them. Make a double batch; it reheats well in the microwave.

Actually a seed rather than a grain, both red and the more common white quinoa are usually available in supermarkets or health food stores. Not only is quinoa high in fiber and healthy nutrients, the protein it supplies is "complete," meaning that it includes all nine essential amino acids, in particular lysine, which is essential for tissue growth and repair and important for growing children.

1	large butternut squash, seeds removed, peeled, cut into 1-inch cubes	5	Tbsp. extra virgin olive oil
1¾	cup water or vegetable stock	1	cup dry red quinoa
1	medium red onion, finely chopped	1	cup toasted pistachios (optional)
	Salt and freshly ground black pepper to taste	½	cup fresh flat-leaf parsley, finely chopped (optional)

Heat oven to 425°F. Toss butternut squash with 2 Tbsp. olive oil, salt, and pepper. Roast in the oven for approximately 30–45 minutes, turning once, until squash has softened and begun to brown. Remove from oven and set aside to cool in pan.

Bring water or stock to a boil in a small pot. Reduce heat and keep at a simmer until ready to use. Toast quinoa in a dry skillet (or whatever you would use to cook rice) on medium-high heat, stirring constantly with a wooden spoon until a nutty aroma rises from the pan (about 2 minutes). When the grain smells toasty, carefully pour the hot liquid slowly into the pan with the quinoa (do this slowly or it will boil over). Add a large pinch of salt, reduce to a simmer over low heat, cover, and cook for about 20 minutes, until water is absorbed. Fluff with a fork and season with salt and freshly ground pepper as desired. Carefully fold in cooled squash, remaining olive oil, and remaining ingredients.

Makes 4–6 servings.

Asian Cabbage Salad

Jean Welsh

1	head of cabbage, finely shredded (or equivalent preshredded)	1	bunch of scallions, chopped
2	packages chicken-flavored ramen noodles (uncooked), broken into pieces	½	cup slivered almonds, toasted until golden brown
1	cup olive oil	5	Tbsp. balsamic vinegar
1	tsp. pepper	1½	tsp. salt
		4	Tbsp. sugar

Mix the cabbage, scallion, noodles, and almonds and set aside. Mix olive oil, balsamic vinegar, salt, pepper, and sugar together. Pour over salad 30 minutes before serving.

Peas with Shallots and Butter

Sanna Delmonico

Especially delicious with fresh peas at their peak in spring.

1	Tbsp. butter	2	shallots, peeled and finely sliced
2	cups fresh peas (about 2 lb. peas in the pods) or frozen peas	¼	cup water
			Salt and fresh ground pepper to taste

Melt butter in a large skillet. Add the shallots and sauté over medium-low heat until translucent, about 3 minutes. Don't let them brown. Add the peas and water, bring to a simmer, cover, and cook until the peas are tender, about 5–7 minutes. Uncover, increase the heat and allow the water to evaporate. Season with salt and pepper and serve hot.

Makes 4–6 servings.

Sesame-Cucumber Salad

Sanna Delmonico

Crisp cucumbers, direct from the garden or local farmer's market, are refreshing in this quick salad. This is the perfect addition to a lunch box.

1	Tbsp. sesame seeds	3	medium cucumbers
4	tsp. rice wine vinegar	1	tsp. sesame oil
	Salt to taste		

Heat the sesame seeds in a small dry (no oil or water) skillet, stirring frequently, until they begin to brown. Remove from heat and let cool. Peel and thinly slice cucumbers. Toss them in a small bowl with the vinegar, oil, and salt and top with toasted sesame seeds.

Makes 4–6 servings.

Homemade Ketchup

Michelle McKenzie

Most store-bought ketchup is loaded with sugar, corn syrup, and preservatives. Luckily, making this favorite condiment from scratch takes relatively little time and can be made in large batches; store in refrigerator, covered, for up to 1 month or in the freezer in an airtight container for up to 5 months. Adjust the spices and sweetness to your and your child's liking.

1	28-oz. can peeled, whole tomatoes	1	medium yellow onion, peeled and quartered
2	cloves garlic, crushed and peeled		
2	Tbsp. honey	½	cup apple cider vinegar
1	cup water	Dash	Tabasco or pinch of cayenne
1	Tbsp. Dijon mustard	Pinch	ground allspice
Pinch	ground cloves	Pinch	ground ginger
Pinch	ground cinnamon		Salt and black pepper

Put tomatoes, onions, garlic, and honey into a blender or food processor and pulse until blended. Add vinegar and 1 cup water and purée until smooth. Transfer to a medium saucepan and add spices except salt and pepper to taste. Cook over low heat, stirring occasionally, for 30–45 minutes, until thick. When done, season to taste with salt and pepper.

Makes 6–8 servings.

Fast, Easy Dinners

Some fast dinners come from crock pots set to cook all day, soups that can be reheated, and casseroles that can be assembled ahead of time and popped in the oven once you arrive home. Most kids like soup, and this is a good way to serve vegetables. If you serve meat, buy thin-sliced cuts so they can be quickly sautéed or marinate pieces cut into serving sizes overnight for grilling at dinnertime. Make sure your dinner also includes vegetables, simply prepared and on the side or included in the mix.

Sausage Soup with Spinach

Martha Meijers

This goes well with a thick slice of fresh whole wheat bread.

½ lb. Italian sausage (or turkey, pork, or chicken sausage)
| medium onion, chopped
| cup brown rice or wild rice, cooked (~½ cup uncooked)
16 oz. low-sodium chicken broth
| tsp. dried or fresh oregano
3 cups torn washed spinach leaves
Salt and pepper to taste

| tsp. olive oil
| clove garlic (optional)
3 cups water
14 oz. diced, crushed, or chopped tomatoes (use 1 lb. fresh chopped tomatoes when available)
½ tsp. dried basil (use 2 tsp. fresh chopped basil when available)
Grated cheese (Parmesan or other aged hard cheese)

Remove sausage casing, if necessary. Sauté sausage and onion in olive oil until the sausage is crumbled and fully cooked and the onions are soft. Drain and remove fat. Add water, tomatoes, and spices and simmer for several minutes. Stir in the cooked rice and torn spinach and taste to see if it needs salt and pepper. Once spinach is soft, serve immediately with grated cheese sprinkled on top or refrigerate and reheat.

Makes 4–5 servings

Slow Cooker Chili

Marion McClain

| lb. lean ground beef, browned, crumbled, and drained of excess fat
1–2 tsp. chili powder
1–2 bay leaves
2 8-oz. cans tomato sauce
| 16-oz. can unseasoned stewed tomatoes

| small onion, chopped
| small shallot, chopped
| tsp. cumin
| tsp. Worcestershire sauce
| 16-oz. can kidney beans, drained
Grated cheddar cheese for topping

Combine all ingredients in a slow cooker and cook on high for 2–3 hours or on low for 6–8 hours. Remove bay leaf. Serve with grated cheddar cheese on top. If you like it hotter, add more chili powder and pepper.

Makes 6–7 servings.

Quick and Easy Vermouth Chicken

Chef Athena Penson

Serve with your favorite pasta or mashed potatoes and steamed vegetables.

2	boneless, skinless chicken breasts	¼	cup flour
1	Tbsp butter	1	Tbsp. olive oil (more if needed)
¼	cup dry vermouth or dry white wine		Salt and pepper to taste
¼	cup chicken broth (more if needed)		

For quick cooking, pound each breast flat to an even thickness of about ⅛–¼ inch. Season with salt and pepper and lightly dredge each piece in the flour. Pat off any excess flour and set aside.

Heat olive oil on medium-high heat in a nonstick sauté pan. Add chicken and sauté until golden on each side, turning chicken *only once*. Cooking time will be 3–4 minutes for each side. Set aside and cover to keep warm.

Take the hot sauté pan off the heat and add the vermouth. Return to the stove top and on a lower heat allow the sauce to start reducing (boil off liquid, leaving a thicker sauce). Stir well to allow all the fond (all the tasty bits and pieces left in the pan) to mix in with the wine to create a tasty sauce. Add the chicken broth, mix well, and then stir in the butter and allow this to reduce further. Add the chicken and cover with the sauce and bring to a boil. Serve immediately.

Tasty Salsa Chicken

Chef Athena Penson

Serve over rice, with black beans and corn on the side. This dish can also be served as an appetizer, over nacho chips topped with sour cream, chopped green onions, and cheddar cheese.

2	boneless, skinless chicken breasts	¼	cup flour
1	Tbsp. butter (optional)	1	Tbsp. olive oil (more if needed)
¼	cup dry vermouth or dry white wine (or substitute chicken broth)		Salt and pepper to taste
½	cup of your favorite salsa (more if you prefer)	¼	cup chicken broth
		¼	cup sharp cheddar cheese, grated

For quick cooking, pound each breast flat to an even thickness of about ⅛–¼ inch (or cut chicken into ½-inch cubes). Season with salt and pepper and lightly dredge each piece in the flour. Pat off any excess flour and set aside.

In a nonstick sauté pan heat the olive oil on medium-high heat. Add chicken and sauté until golden on each side, turning chicken *only once*. Cooking time will be 3–4 minutes for each side. Set aside and cover to keep warm.

Take the hot sauté pan off the heat and add the vermouth. Return to the stove top and on a lower heat allow the sauce to start reducing (boil off liquid, leaving a thicker sauce). Stir well to allow all the fond (all the tasty bits and pieces left on the pan) to mix in with wine and create a tasty sauce. Add the chicken broth, mix well, and then stir in the butter and allow this to reduce further, 1–2 minutes. Add the salsa and bring to a boil. Add the chicken back to the pan, cover with the sauce, and bring to a boil again. Sprinkle with grated cheese.

Chicken Souvlaki

Chef Athena Penson

Marinate chicken the night before and place in refrigerator until ready to prepare the meal.

1	lb. boneless, skinless chicken breasts	1–2	garlic cloves
2	tsp. dried oregano	1½	tsp. cumin, ground
1	tsp. paprika	3	Tbsp. lemon juice
½	extra virgin olive oil	1½	tsp. salt
1	tsp. pepper		Bamboo skewers for grilling
4	Pieces whole wheat pita bread		(unless you sauté the chicken)
	Fresh tomatoes		Lettuce, shredded
	Tzatziki sauce (see recipe below)		

Cut the chicken breasts into 1-inch cubes and set aside. In a bowl, prepare marinade by mixing garlic, oregano, cumin, paprika, lemon juice, olive oil, salt, and pepper until well blended. Pour marinade over chicken, mix, cover, and let it marinate for 30 minutes or overnight in refrigerator.

Soak skewers in water for at least 30 minutes. Place chicken pieces on skewers and grill (or sauté) chicken until cooked all the way through. While chicken is cooking, warm pita bread in oven. To assemble, place chicken on or in pita bread and top with tomatoes, lettuce, and tzatziki. Fold, eat, and enjoy!

Makes 4 servings.

Tzatziki

Chef Athena Penson

32	oz. authentic Greek yogurt (or plain yogurt), strained cucumber	½	tsp. salt and pepper (or more to taste)
1	cucumber	¼	tsp. olive oil (or more to tasste)
1–2	large garlic cloves (or more to taste), crushed	¼	tsp. lemon juice (or more to taste)
2	tsp. dried dill (use 1 Tbsp. chopped fresh dill when available)		

To strain yogurt, place a large piece of cheesecloth or paper towel in a sieve (or colander) over a bowl. Add yogurt. Fold the draped edges of the cheesecloth (if used) over the yogurt, and place in refrigerator for 1–2 hours (the longer you leave it, the thicker the yogurt will get). Place a small plate on top of the yogurt to aid in the drainage of excess water.

Peel, seed, and coarsely grate the cucumber and place in a sieve (or colander) or wrap in chesecloth and squeeze out as much water as possible.

Place all ingredients in a bowl and mix well. Chill in the refrigerator for at least 2 hours. Season to taste with salt.

Pecan-Crusted Chicken Fingers

Chef Virginia Willis

Panko has fewer calories, less sodium, and more fiber than regular breadcrumbs.

1	lb. pound boneless, skinless chicken breasts, cut into ½" x 2" strips	1	cup whole wheat flour
3	large egg whites, lightly beaten	¾	cup panko (Japanese-style) or unseasoned breadcrumbs
¾	cup finely chopped pecans		Coarse salt and freshly ground black pepper

Heat oven to 400°F. Place a baking rack over a baking sheet. Set aside.

Place the flour in a shallow dish and season with salt and pepper. Place egg whites in a separate shallow dish and season with salt and pepper. Combine the breadcrumbs and pecans in a shallow dish. Add salt and pepper.

Dredge chicken strips in flour, shaking off excess, dip in egg white mixture, and then coat with breadcrumb mixture. Place the chicken strips on the prepared rack. Bake for 20–25 minutes until cooked golden brown and the juices run clear when the chicken is pierced with a knife.

Makes 4 servings.

Mexican Chicken Soup

Miriam Vos

3	chicken thighs	4	cups water or low-sodium chicken broth
1	28-oz. can diced tomatoes		
3	garlic cloves, minced	1	large onion, chopped
¼	cup chopped fresh cilantro	1½	cups frozen corn
	Salt	½	fresh lime, squeezed for juice
	Optional toppings:		
	Chopped fresh cilantro		
	Coarsely crushed corn tortilla chips		
	Sour cream or yogurt		
	Avocado, chopped into bite-sized pieces		

In large pot, combine chicken, water, tomatoes, garlic, onion, and cilantro. Simmer on medium-high for 1 hour or until chicken is tender. Remove chicken from pot and set on a plate to cool. When cool, remove the skin and remove meat from bones. Discard skin and bones. Chop meat coarsely, return to soup pot, add corn, and simmer for about 10 minutes. Salt to taste. If soup is too thick, add more water to taste. After removing from heat, add lime juice. Serve in large bowls and pass around desired toppings.

Makes 10–12 cups of soup.

Chicken "Long Rice"

Chef Amy Ponzoli

If you buy an extra stalk or two of lemon grass in the early spring, it is very easy to grow. Set it in the window in a glass with an inch or so of water for a few days and then stick it into a small pot of soil either outside or inside if it's still freezing at night. If you keep the soil moist, the grass will root and start to shoot new leaves up from the center. Once you move it to a bigger pot or plant it in the garden, it takes off. That way, you'll have fresh lemon grass just outside the back door all summer long!

6	oz. bean thread noodles		1	oz. sesame oil
1	oz. canola oil		1	lb. boneless, skinless chicken
1	oz. lemon grass, minced			breasts, cut in strips
1	oz. ginger, minced		2	garlic cloves, minced
½	cup low-sodium chicken broth		1	oz. low-sodium soy sauce
1	tsp. salt (optional)		3	Tbsp. toasted sesame seeds
2	oz. green onions, sliced		½	cup orange sections

Boil noodles until just soft, drain, place in a large serving bowl, coat with sesame oil, and chill. Heat canola oil in pan and add chicken, cooking a few minutes until half-way done. Add lemon grass, ginger, garlic, broth, and soy sauce. Continue to cook until chicken is done, adding salt. Mix chicken into noodles. Serve topped with sesame seeds, green onions, and orange sections.

Makes 4–6 servings.

Mashed Potato and Meat Casserole

Christine Malek

The mashed potatoes in this casserole are dairy free, so it's great for kids who are lactose intolerant.

6	large white potatoes	I	large onion, chopped
I	Tbsp. canola oil	I	lb. lean ground beef (93% lean)
	Salt and pepper	½	tsp. cinnamon
I	egg, beaten	½	cup unseasoned bread crumbs
I	Tbsp. olive oil		(can make your own from whole-grain bread)

Wash and peel potatoes, cut into chunks. In a large pot boil potatoes in water. While potatoes cook, sauté chopped onion in canola oil, add ground beef and cook until done. Stir in salt and pepper to taste; add cinnamon. Set aside. When potatoes are tender, drain thoroughly and mash with salt to taste and add egg. Grease or spray with cooking spray a 9 × 13 inch dish and spread half of potato mixture on bottom. Spread all of meat mixture on top. Layer remaining potato mixture next. Sprinkle breadcrumbs on top and drizzle olive oil over breadcrumbs. Bake at 350°F for 20 minutes or until heated through and browned on top. It may be necessary to broil casserole for 1–2 minutes to brown before serving.

Makes 12 servings.

Spaghetti Pies

Ellen Stokes

These freeze beautifully. You can make these in disposable pie pans or in smaller pans.

16	oz. whole-grain spaghetti	6	Tbsp. butter
1¼	cups Parmesan cheese	3	eggs, beaten
	Nonstick cooking spray	3	lb. lean ground beef (93% lean)
1	cup finely chopped onion	1	Tbsp. canola oil
2	15-oz. cans tomato sauce	2	6-oz. cans tomato paste
2	tsp. sugar	⅓	cup water
1	Tbsp. dried oregano		Garlic salt, dried basil, and
2	cups fat-free sour cream		pepper to taste
8	oz. shredded mozzarella cheese		

Boil water in large pot. Add spaghetti, cook until *al dente* (still firm, not soggy), drain. Stir in butter, Parmesan cheese, and eggs. Chop spaghetti mixture into small pieces using two knives; divide mixture three ways into three 9-inch pie pans that have been sprayed with nonstick cooking spray (or lightly greased with oil). Place spaghetti in pie pans. Form mixture into a "crust" in each pan, pressing down firmly in bottom and along sides. Set aside to cool.

Heat oil in large skillet. Cook ground beef and onion. Stir in tomato sauce, tomato paste, sugar, water, and other seasonings. Continue cooking until mixture is heated. Spread sour cream divided three ways over spaghetti crusts. Fill pies with meat sauce. Cover with shredded mozzarella. Bake at 350°F for 30 minutes or freeze immediately. Thaw frozen pie before baking.

Makes three 9-inch pies; 18 servings.

Kale Soup

Jolene Vos

Adjust the proportions of ingredients in this hearty soup to your liking. Any leftovers freeze very well.

1	medium onion	5	garlic cloves
1	bunch kale, with stems	1	Tbsp. canola oil
	(cooks down to 1½ cups)	1	quart chicken broth
2	medium potatoes		(use low-sodium or homemade
3	medium carrots		broth if available)
2	cups cooked white beans	½–1	lb. reduced-fat Polish sausage
	(canned navy or Great Northern		(Kielbasa), cut in small pieces
	beans can be used, drain before		(low sodium if available)
	adding to soup)		
	Salt and pepper to taste		

Chop onion, garlic, and kale. Cook in canola oil in 2-quart heavy saucepan until almost tender. Add chicken broth. Wash potatoes, peel, and chop potatoes. Add to broth along with washed and chopped carrots. Cook soup until vegetables are tender. Add white beans and chopped sausage. Season to taste.

Make about 12 cups of soup.

Greek Meatballs

Julia Kitromelides

Make meatballs the previous day and bake prior to serving. Baked meatballs easily freeze and can be frozen for later use.

1	lb. lean ground beef	1	cup unseasoned bread crumbs
½	onion, minced	2	eggs, beaten
½	tsp. salt	⅛	tsp. pepper
¼	tsp. cinnamon	1	Tbsp. dried mint
1	tsp. dried oregano	1	clove garlic, minced
	Olive oil cooking spray	2	Tbsp. extra virgin olive oil

Combine all ingredients thoroughly (except olive oil spray and extra virgin olive oil). Make small (1-inch) balls from mixture. Refrigerate meat balls for at least one hour. Preheat oven to 400°F. Spray two 8 × 10–inch pans with olive oil cooking spray. Place meatballs evenly in each pan. Drizzle olive oil on the meatballs. Bake for 20 minutes. Turn over meatballs; bake an additional 20 minutes or until crispy and brown. Serve with Greek yogurt and pita bread.

Makes 5 servings (about 30 meatballs).

Warm Penne with Fresh Tomatoes and Basil

Xiomara Hinson

1¼	lb. dried whole wheat penne pasta	5	very ripe plum tomatoes
½	yellow pepper	1	small bunch fresh basil
4	Tbsp. extra virgin olive oil	2	Tbsp. pesto
	Salt and pepper to taste		

Cook pasta according to directions on package. While pasta cooks, chop tomatoes and yellow pepper. Wash basil. Remove leaves from stems; discard stems. Chop leaves finely. When pasta is cooked *al dente* (still firm, not soggy), drain thoroughly. Toss with tomatoes, pepper, basil, and olive oil. Add pesto sauce to mixture. Season with salt and pepper. Serve immediately.

Tomato Meatball Soup

Miriam Vos

3½	cups water	1	28-oz. can diced or crushed
1	lb. ground beef		tomatoes
	(ground round or chuck)	⅓	cup barley
1	large onion, chopped	1	cup chopped celery leaves and
2	carrots, chopped into 1-inch pieces		2 celery stalks (use the heart of
1	bay leaf		the celery)
1	tsp. fresh ground pepper	1	tsp. salt

In a large soup pot, bring water and tomatoes to boil. Mix ¼ teaspoon black pepper and ¼ teaspoon salt into ground beef and shape into ¾ inch meatballs (bite size). Add meatballs to boiling liquid and then reduce to simmer. Add remaining ingredients. Simmer for ~1 hour or until barley and vegetables are tender. You can add extra vegetables to this depending on what is in season and your family's preferences. For a thicker soup decrease the water, for thinner increase. Season with additional salt and pepper to taste before serving. Serve with a slice of hearty whole-grain bread and green salad.

Makes 10 servings

Swiss Chard Quiche

Jolene Vos

Swiss chard has brilliant green leaves and white stalks that are highly nutritious and flavorful. It's related to spinach but has a slightly bitter and salty flavor that grows on you.

8 Tbsp. butter	¼ cup milk (or more if needed)
½ tsp. salt	1 bunch Swiss chard (or other greens, like spinach) washed and chopped (about 5 cups)
1 onion, chopped	
4 eggs	
½ cup milk	1 tsp. salt
¼ cup sour cream	1 cup grated Gruyere, Emmental, or Swiss cheese
¼ tsp. pepper	
1½ cups whole wheat flour	

For crust, cut 6 Tbsp. butter into flour and ½ teaspoon salt in medium mixing bowl. Work with fingers until it becomes coarse crumbs. Add ¼ cup milk. Mix with hands and form ball. Let it "rest" in refrigerator for 20–30 minutes while you prepare filling.

For filling, cook onion and chopped Swiss chard stems in 2 Tbsp. butter. Add chopped greens and cook until wilted. In a separate bowl, beat eggs and mix in ½ cup milk, sour cream, salt, and pepper.

Roll out the crust on a floured surface and fit into pie pan. Spread shredded cheese in pie crust. Spread cooked onions and greens over the cheese. Pour milk and egg mixture over the greens. Bake in oven preheated to 425°F for 20 minutes. Reduce heat to 375°F and bake for an additional 30 minutes or until the top of quiche is golden.

The quiche can be frozen before baking. To bake a frozen quiche, place in preheated 425°F oven for 50 minutes. Reduce heat to 375°F, and bake another 30 minutes until done.

Panko Chicken Strips

Clare Aslaksen

Panko has fewer calories, less sodium, and more fiber than regular breadcrumbs.

2	lb. boneless skinless chicken breasts	½	cup low-fat plain yogurt
¼	tsp. garlic, minced or crushed	1	cup panko (Japanese-style) or
¼	cup grated Parmesan cheese		regular breadcrumbs
1	tsp. parsley or other favorite herb		

Cut chicken breasts into strips. Mix yogurt and garlic in a container that has a lid. Place chicken strips into the yogurt mixture and coat the strips. Place lid on container and marinate in refrigerator for several hours or overnight. Preheat oven to 450°F. Mix the breadcrumbs, Parmesan cheese, and parsley in a shallow bowl or plate. Coat the strips on one side only with the breadcrumb mixture. Place on a cookie sheet lined with parchment paper, breadcrumb side up. Bake for 15 minutes.

Turkey Picadillo Sandwiches

Chef Libby Stewart

1	tsp. olive oil	1	large onion, finely chopped
1	large red bell pepper, chopped	¾	lb. ground turkey
2	cloves garlic, chopped or crushed	1	Tbsp. chili powder
2	tsp. ground cumin	¼	tsp. ground cinnamon
1	16-oz. can tomato sauce	3	Tbsp. balsamic vinegar
⅓	cup golden raisins, chopped	¼	cup pimiento-stuffed green
¼	tsp. salt		olives, chopped
¼	tsp. pepper	4	soft whole wheat sandwich buns

Heat a nonstick skillet over medium heat. Add the oil, onion, and bell pepper and cook for 5 minutes, or until softened, stirring occasionally. Increase the heat to medium-high and add the turkey. Cook for 5 minutes, breaking up the meat with a spoon until it is no longer pink. Stir in the remaining ingredients, except buns, and cook for 15 minutes or until thickened, stirring occasionally. Spoon the meat mixture onto the bottom halves of the buns, dividing evenly. Cover with the bun tops.

Makes 4 servings.

Whole Wheat Pasta with Chard and Olives

Sanna Delmonico

Hearty and satisfying, this pasta dish comes together in less than 30 minutes. Add some sliced fruit and crusty bread, and you have a meal.

1 lb. whole wheat penne (or other short pasta shape)	1 Tbsp. olive oil
4 cloves garlic, thinly sliced	1 bunch Swiss chard, washed and chopped (about 5 cups)
Salt and pepper to taste	Pinch red pepper (optional)
2–3 Tbsp. olive tapenade (or finely chopped black olives)	Grated Parmesan cheese

Bring a large pot of salted water to a rolling boil. Add the pasta and cook according to package directions, until just done. Meanwhile, heat the olive oil in a large skillet over medium heat. Add sliced garlic, and sauté for a few minutes, until garlic begins to turn golden brown. Add chopped chard and ¼ cup water, cover, reduce heat, and cook until the chard is tender, about 7 minutes. Uncover and pour off any excess water.

When pasta is cooked, drain it well and add to the skillet. Add salt, pepper, and red pepper to taste, along with a splash of olive oil. Toss with the olive tapenade and serve topped with Parmesan cheese.

Makes 4–6 servings.

One Good Pea Soup

Eden Myers

When I first served this soup, my daughter took a spoonful, tasted it, and declared, "That's one good pea soup!" This is a low-fat, high-fiber, high-flavor dish that almost every kid likes. Feel free to substitute—water for wine, ham for lamb, parsnip for potato—to suit your taste and the contents of your cupboard.

½	lb. smoked leg of lamb	2	Tbsp. olive oil
1	medium onion, diced	1	cup white wine
½	rutabaga, peeled and diced	½	large potato, peeled and diced
1½	cup dried green split peas		

Sauté leg of lamb slices in olive oil in a large soup pot on medium heat until browned. Add onion, and sauté until translucent. Remove lamb and onion from pot. Add wine, mixing it with all the browned bits scraped off the bottom of the pot. Add rutabaga and enough water to cover. Simmer on low for 10 minutes. Add potato, peas, and lamb-onion mixture to the pot, add water to cover, and simmer on low for another 20 minutes, adding water if soup becomes too thick. When finished cooking and peas are soft, remove some of the meat and vegetables, and puree the rest in a blender or with a hand mixer in the pot. Add the reserved pieces back to the smooth soup. Add more hot water if soup becomes too thick.

Makes 6–8 servings.

Crockpot Lamb Shanks

Eden Myers

This recipe has, in my son's words, "Everything I like and nothing I don't!" I like it because it is easy, healthy, and tasty—and did I mention easy? Substitute 1 can of tomato sauce plus 1 garlic clove and 1 Tbsp. honey for the brand-name spaghetti sauce.

2	lbs. cross-cut lamb hindshanks, cut into 8 pieces ("osso bucco" style)	1	28-oz. can diced tomatoes
1	onion, chopped	½	bottle dry white wine
½	jar Ragu Roasted Garlic spaghetti sauce	½	lb. baby carrots
		½	cup diced celery

Put all ingredients in crock pot and heat on low for 6 hours. Serve over cooked whole wheat penne or brown rice.

Makes 4 servings.

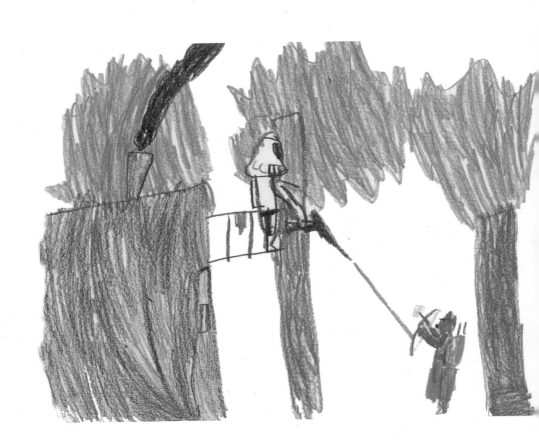

Healthy Snack Ideas

The best snacks are those that combine fiber with protein. This combination is filling, healthy, and gives you a great opportunity to get creative. Sources of fiber are fruits, vegetables, and whole grains. Cheese, yogurt, and nut butters are kid-friendly sources of protein. Mix and match these fiber and protein rich foods for a healthy snack your child will love.

Cynthia Chandler Kennedy, MS, RD, LD, CDM, contributed these tips and the following snack ideas. Keep colors in mind. Children like to pick up attractive foods and handle their own food. Try cutting fruit into bite-sized segments and serving on a colorful plate. On the side, have a small dish of peanut butter, strawberry-flavored cream cheese thinned with milk to dipping consistency, or honey with a honey server that can be lightly dripped onto the fruit. Look for unusual fruits like starfruits and figs that you may not have tried yet.

Fruits and Vegetables	Dips and Spreads	Snacks, Cereals, and Grains
Squash or zucchini circles	Almond butter, cashew	Granola
Broccoli or cauliflower	butter, peanut butter	Whole wheat crackers
"trees"	Plain or vanilla yogurt	with pieces of cheese
Orange slices	Black bean dip	Kashi cereal
Apple or pear slices	Hummus	Whole wheat cookies
Berries	Salad dressing	Peanut butter sandwich
Peaches		made with whole
Bananas		wheat bread
Raisins		Nuts
Cucumber slices		Whole-grain crackers
Cherry tomatoes		Whole-grain pita bread
Tomato wedges		Whole-grain breakfast
Carrot sticks		cereals
Green or red pepper slices		Whole wheat tortillas
Avocados		
Olives		
Snow or sugar snap peas		

Snack ideas:

- Wasa crispbread spread with 1 Tbsp. cream cheese and 2 tsp. peach or mango chutney or any type of jelly. Eat open faced after school with a glass of milk.
- Stuff a fig or date with cream cheese for a bite-sized snack that is sweet and full of fiber.

☺ Try freezing a banana or grapes—great on hot summer days.

☺ Make a smoothie by blending a cup of frozen yogurt, a handful of blueberries and strawberries, and a drizzle of honey.

☺ Cook flatbread topped with tomato sauce and parmesan or other cheese (can add cooked chicken strips) under broiler for 2 minutes until cheese is melted.

☺ Make your own "trail mix." I like to call it the "car mix" as we often are eating in the car.

"On the Way to School" Mix

Cynthia Chandler Kennedy, MS, RD, LD, CDM

2	Turkish figs, dates, or raisins (chopped if needed)	2	Tbsp. walnuts, chopped
¼	cup toasted oat bran cereal or your favorite high-fiber cereal		

Mix ingredients and put in zip lock bag for snacking. This could also be used as a morning snack or put in the lunchbox, paired with some apple slices and peanut butter.

Peanut Butter–Banana Curls

Chef Carmen Capello

½	cup peanut butter	⅓	cup vanilla organic yogurt
1	Tbsp. orange juice	2	ripe, organic bananas, sliced
4	8-inch whole wheat tortillas	2	Tbsp. honey-crunch wheat germ
¼	tsp. ground cinnamon		

Combine peanut butter and yogurt, stirring until smooth. Drizzle juice over bananas; toss gently to coat. Spread about 3 Tbsp. peanut butter mixture over each tortilla, leaving a ½-inch border. Arrange about ⅓ cup banana slices in a single layer over peanut butter mixture. Combine wheat germ and cinnamon; sprinkle evenly over banana slices. Roll up. Slice each roll into 6 pieces.

Makes 6 4-piece servings.

Snack Mix

Chef Amy Ponzoli

½ cup Kix cereal
½ cup Wheat or Rice Chex cereal
¼ cup flax seed
¼ cup honey
Nonstick cooking spray
1 cup dried fruit (raisins, dried cranberries, chopped dried pineapple, etc.)

½ cup Cheerios cereal
½ cup whole oats
2 Tbsp. peanut butter
1 egg white, beaten
1 cup pretzel sticks

Preheat oven to 325°F. In a bowl, mix together first 8 ingredients. Make sure egg white is beaten thoroughly before adding to mix. Spray cookie sheet with non-stick cooking spray and pour ingredients onto pan in a single layer. Bake until lightly toasted and dry. When cool, toss with pretzel sticks and fruit.

Makes 5–6 cups

*Above all, let your child
make a mess in the kitchen
and cook with you.*

Spacefood

Chef Amy Ponzoli

2 quart-size zip lock bags
2 Tbsp. peanut butter
2 Tbsp. ground flax seeds

4 whole graham crackers (8 squares)
2 tsp. honey

Put 2 whole graham crackers in each bag. Crumble the crackers into sand consistency. Divide peanut butter, flax seeds, and honey equally into the bags and mix thoroughly with the graham cracker crumbs. Once mixed, squeeze all ingredients into one corner of the bag. Using scissors snip off a small corner of each bag. Have your kids cover the hole with their lips and squeeze the snack into their mouths—just like astronauts!

Makes 2 snacks.

Worms on a Leaf

Chef Amy Ponzoli

4	large outer romaine lettuce leaves, cleaned and dried	1½	cups cooked buckwheat soba or whole wheat spaghetti noodles, coated in sesame oil
½	red pepper, cut into strips		
1	carrot, grated	2	cooked and seasoned boneless chicken breasts, cut into strips
4	oz. Teriyaki sauce (for dipping)		

Arrange ¼ of all ingredients into the center of 1 romaine leaf and roll to resemble an egg roll. Use a toothpick to hold if needed. Repeat 3 times. These can be made ahead of time. To store, wrap a moist paper towel over assembled leaves and cover tightly.

Makes 4 "leaves."

Roll-Ups

Jill Nussinow, MS, RD (The Veggie Queen)

These are nothing more than tortillas that have been filled, rolled, and sliced. Many kids like them better than sandwiches. Roll-ups are limited only by your imagination. Think about adding grated carrots, sprouts, shredded apple, or your child's favorite fruit or vegetable.

Bean Roll-Ups

1	whole wheat tortilla (any size)	¼	cup (or more) refried beans, warmed
2	Tbsp. salsa or sliced tomato		
2	Tbsp. grated cheese (optional)		

Spread refried beans on tortilla. Top with salsa or tomato and cheese (optional). Roll tortilla tightly. Cut into slices and stand upright.

For nut butter and fruit spread roll-ups, use 2 Tbsp. peanut, almond, cashew, or soy butter instead of beans and use fruit spread instead of salsa. Roll and cut in the same way.

Black Bean Hummus, Turkey, Avocado, and Tomato Roll-Ups

Chef David Bressler

Store hummus in the refrigerator for up to 1 week.

3	cups cooked black beans	3	cups cooked lima or butter beans
½	Tbsp. cumin	3	Tbsp. sesame tahini
3	Tbsp. lime juice	½	cup olive oil
	Salt and pepper, to taste	¼	lb. sliced deli turkey
1	avocado, thinly sliced	1	vine ripe tomato, diced
1	tortilla—whole wheat, spinach, or other flavor		

Combine beans, cumin, tahini, lime juice, and oil in a food processor and blend well. Add salt and pepper to taste. Cover and chill.

To make roll-ups, spread black bean hummus on tortilla from end to end. On the lower quarter of the tortilla, place turkey, tomatoes, and avocado. Roll tortilla tight. Use a dab of hummus to seal the tortilla. Slice in ½-inch slices to create pinwheels.

Tofu Fruit Smoothie

Jill Nussinow, MS, RD (The Veggie Queen)

Smoothie will keep in the refrigerator for up to 3 days. If it separates, shake to mix. If you prefer, use 12–16 ounces of yogurt instead of tofu.

1	cup frozen fruit of any type; berries work especially well	¾	cup any fruit juice, such as apple or orange
½	box (12.3 oz.) Silken lite firm or extra firm tofu		

Put all ingredients into blender and blend until smooth. Serve chilled.

Makes 2 cups.

Homemade Granola Bars

Laura Martin

2	cups rolled oats	1	teaspoon cinnamon
½	cup chopped nuts, such walnuts, almonds, pecans	½	cup chopped dried fruits, raisins, figs, dates, "fruit bits"
3	Tbsp. vegetable oil, plus enough to grease baking pan	¼	cup natural sweetener, such as honey or maple syrup (if you use brown rice syrup or barley malt syrup, use ⅓ cup)
2	Tbsp. fruit juice, such as apple, pear, or white grape		
1	banana, mashed	1	egg, beaten (can omit egg and use 1½ mashed bananas)

Preheat oven to 350°F. Grease 9-inch-square baking pan with oil (or line with parchment paper). Mix together oats, nuts, fruit, and cinnamon in a bowl. In another bowl, combine 3 Tbsp. oil, sweetener, and juice. Mix well and then add egg and mashed banana. (Note: If you grease the measuring cup before you pour the sweetener in, you'll get a more accurate measurement and clean up will be easier.) Blend this mixture into the oat/nut mix and blend well. Press mixture into the prepared pan. Bake for 20–25 minutes. When cool, cut into squares.

Dippin' Frozen Berries

Clare Aslasken

Why use chopsticks? Your children will learn dexterity, experience how a different culture eats, and they will eat more slowly!

1	lb. any berries that are in season	1	cup plain yogurt
1	tsp. almond or vanilla extract		

Wash and drain berries, removing stems and leaves and discarding any mushy berries. Remove hulls if using strawberries. Place berries in a single layer on a large baking sheet with edges (so the berries will not roll off or stick together) and place in freezer. Alternatively, use a smaller container and either freeze smaller portions or arrange in multiple layers and break berries apart after freezing.

Whisk together yogurt and extract. Serve the frozen berries and dip with chopsticks.

Freeze berries ahead of time to use later by "vacuum packing" them. Put the berries in a zip lock bag with a drinking straw inside the bag, zipping it as closed as possible with the straw protruding from the bag. Using the straw, suck the air out of the bag, pinch the straw, then remove the straw quickly and close bag tightly.

Lunchbox Ladybugs on a Stick

Clare Aslasken

Celery stalks   Low-fat Laughing Cow cheese
Ground almonds   Dried cranberries

Wash celery stalks and pat dry. Spread the cheese on 3-inch pieces of celery stalk. Sprinkle ground almonds on top of each piece. Decorate with the cranberries as "ladybugs."

Whole Wheat Tortilla Chips and Apple Salsa

Clare Aslaksen

1	tsp. ground cumin	½	tsp. salt
½	tsp. chili powder (optional—add if your child like things a little spicy)	½	cup olive oil
		2	apples, favorite variety
4	large whole wheat tortillas	1	red pepper
3	large tomatoes	⅓	cup chopped cilantro
1	green pepper	¼	tsp. salt
1	Tbsp. raspberry or apple cider vinegar		

Mix cumin, salt, and, if desired, chili powder in the olive oil. Brush mixture lightly on the 4 tortillas. Slice each tortilla into 8 "pizza slices." Place on baking pan and bake at 350°F until golden, about 20 minutes.

Core and finely chop apples. Core and chop tomatoes and place in strainer and drain for about 5 minutes. Core and finely chop peppers. Combine apples, tomotoes, peppers, cilantro, vinegar, and salt in a bowl. Refrigerate for 1 hour (or longer) to combine flavors, and serve with homemade tortilla chips.

Resources

Physical Activity

YMCA National (www.ymca.net) will help you find your closest YMCA center and has great ideas on how to play with your kids.

Boys & Girls Clubs of America (www.bgca.org) will help you find the local site for after-school recreation and activities.

www.kidnetic.com is a noncommercial site (no advertising) that promotes active kids sponsored by the International Food Information Council. Under the "fitness" tabs this site lists lots of great ideas for your child to be active.

www.girlpower.gov/default.aspx is an encouraging and motivating site for girls with sections on sports and fitness and on having a healthy body image aimed at 9- to 13-year-old girls. Sponsored by the U.S. Department of Health and Human Services.

www.Bam.gov is a Centers for Disease Control–sponsored site for children and teachers of children, with a fun activity calendar where your child can log in all their new activities . . . including cleaning their rooms!

Max's Magical Delivery Fit for Kids: A DVD for Parents and Kids! is a fun video that explains the connections between food, physical activity, and energy. It's available free from the U.S Department of Health and Human Services, via an electronic order form at www.ahrq.gov/child/dvdobesity.htm.

Time-Scout Monitor is an easy-to-use product that helps parents control the amount of screen time for children. Plug a device, such as a television, video game player or computer, into the Time-Scout's lock and "let the box be the bad guy, not you." www.time-scout.com

The Mother's Almanac, Revised, by Marguerite Kelly and Elia Parsons (Broadway Books, 2001) contains projects and recipes you can do with your children that create a fun and active childhood.

www.nflrush.com/health has some fun ideas to inspire the child (and/or parent) who loves football to be more active. My review of the site suggests that some monitoring would be necessary because it also links to video games and areas for ad lib fan comments.

Healthy Eating

In Defense of Food: An Eater's Manifesto by Michael Pollan (Penguin, 2008) will get you thinking about "food" versus "food products." His philosophy: "Eat food. Not too much. Mostly plants." This book tackles the issues with our food industry, marketing industry, and nutrition science industry.

Your Child's Weight: Helping Without Harming, Birth through Adolescence and **How to Get Your Child to Eat . . . But Not Too Much** by Ellyn Satter, MS, RD, LCSW, BCD, offer wisdom on feeding children. More information is at www.EllynSatter.com.

The Fattening of America: How the Economy Makes Us Fat, If It Matters, and What to Do About It by Eric A. Finkelstein and Laurie Zuckerman (Wiley, 2008) will help you understand more about how our society drives many aspects of the obesity epidemic.

Simpler Living, Compassionate Life: A Christian Perspective edited by Michael Schut (Living the Good News, 1999) is a wonderful collection of essays that covers some important issues that we all share (not enough time, money, peace?).

www.williams-sonoma.com has small Siena Tumblers juice glasses.

www.cdc.gov/nccdphp/dnpa/healthyweight/healthy_eating/energy_density.htm provides helpful information from the Centers for Disease Control and Prevention focuses on how you can reduce the "density" of your food by adding vegetables and cutting fat in your favorite foods.

www.mypyramid.gov from the U.S. Department of Agriculture can help you use food groups to create menu plans for your family for a day or a week and has ways to track your eating habits.

Cooking and Growing Food

Simply in Season by Mary Beth Lind and Cathleen Hockman-Wert (Herald Press, 2005) is a cookbook of whole-grain and vegetable-filled recipes.

The Moosewood Restaurant Cooks at Home: Fast and Easy Recipes for Any Day by Moosewood Collective (Fireside, 1994) features vegetarian recipes with speedy preparation.

Fast Food My Way by Jacques Pepin (Houghton Mifflin Harcourt, 2004) is written by a master chef who takes on the challenge of helping you provide super-fast, tasty meals.

The Junior Leagues' Kids in the Kitchen program (www.kidsinthekitchen.org) features ideas for involving children in food preparation plus many recipes and fitness ideas.

More-with-Less Cookbook, 25th edition, by Doris Janzen Longcare (Herald Press, 2003) has commentaries by Mennonites on how to eat healthier while consuming fewer of the world's resources, with lots of high-fiber, legume- and vegetable-based recipes.

From Asparagus to Zucchini: A Guide to Cooking Farm-Fresh Seasonal Produce by the Madison Area Community Supported Agriculture Coalition (Jones Books, 2004).

The Organic Garden: A Practical Guide to Natural Gardens, from Planning and Planting to Harvesting and Maintaining by Christine and Michael Lavelle (Anness Publishing, 2003)

Territorial Seed Company (www.territorialseed.com), **Seeds of Change** (www.seedsofchange.com), and **Johnny's Seeds** (www.johnnyseeds.com) are sources of seeds for starting a home garden.

www.localharvest.org, www.biodynamics.com/csa, and **www.local organics.org** are sites that have information about community-supported agriculture and farms and list farmer's markets by geographical location.

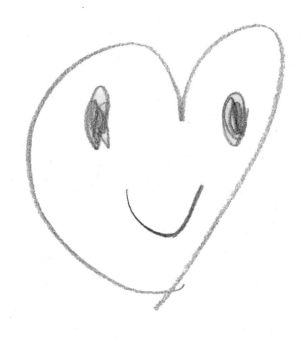

References

1. Olshansky S, Passaro D, Hershow R, et al.: A potential decline in life expectancy in the United States in the 21st century. *N Engl J Med* 352:1138–45, 2005.
2. *Childhood Obesity in the United States: Facts and Figures.* Institute of Medicine of the National Academies, 2004. http://www.iom.edu/ Object.File/Master/22/606/FINALfactsandfigures2.pdf
3. Verhulst SL, Rooman R, Van Gaal L, De Backer W, Desager K: Is sleep-disordered breathing an additional risk factor for the metabolic syndrome in obese children and adolescents? *Int J Obes* (Lond). 33(1):8–13, 2008.
4. McKenzie SA, Bhattacharya A, Sureshkumar R, et al.: Which obese children should have a sleep study? *Respir Med* 102(11):1581–85, 2008
5. Perron AD, Miller MD, Brady WJ: Orthopedic pitfalls in the ED: slipped capital femoral epiphysis. *Am J Emerg Med* 20(5):484–87, 2002.
6. Van Vlierberghe L, Braet C, Goossens L, Mels S: Psychiatric disorders and symptom severity in referred versus non-referred overweight children and adolescents. *Eur Child Adolesc Psychiatry*. Advanced online pub 20 Sept 2008.
7. Gibson LY, Byrne SM, Blair E, Davis EA, Jacoby P, Zubrick SR: Clustering of psychosocial symptoms in overweight children. *Aust N Z J Psychiatry* 42(2):118–25, 2008.
8. Anderson SE, Cohen P, Naumova EN, Jacques PF, Must A: Adolescent obesity and risk for subsequent major depressive disorder and anxiety disorder: prospective evidence. *Psychosom Med* 69(8):740–47, 2007.
9. Li Y, Dai Q, Jackson JC, Zhang J: Overweight is associated with decreased cognitive functioning among school-age children and adolescents. *Obesity (Silver Spring)* 16(8):1809–15, 2008.
10. Hillman CH, Erickson KI, Kramer AF: Be smart, exercise your heart: exercise effects on brain and cognition. *Nat Rev Neurosci* 9(1):58–65, 2008.

11. Adams R, Bukowski W: Peer victimization as a predictor of depression and body mass index in obese and non-obese adolescents. *J Child Psychol Psychiatry* 49(8):858–66, 2008.

12. Raskauskas J, Stoltz A: Identifying and intervening in relational aggression. *J Sch Nurs* 20:209–15, 2004.

13. Lampl M, Thompson A: Growth chart curves do not describe individual growth biology. *Am J Human Biol* 19:643–53, 2007.

14. Whitaker R, Wright J, Pepe M, Seidel K, Dietz W: Predicting obesity in young adulthood from childhood and parental obesity. *N Engl J Med* 337(13):869–73, 1997.

15. Roberts S, Savage J, Coward W, Chew B, Lucas A: Energy expenditure and intake in infants born to lean and overweight mothers. *N Engl J Med* 318(8):461–66, 1988.

16. Ravelli G, Stein Z, Susser M: Obesity in young men after famine exposure in utero and early infancy. *N Engl J Med* 295:349–53, 1976.

17. Boney C, Verma A, Tucker R, Vohr B: Metabolic syndrome in childhood: association with birth weight, maternal obesity, and gestational diabetes mellitus. *Pediatrics* 115:e290–96, 2005.

18. Rising R, Lifshitz F: Lower energy expenditures in infants from obese biological mothers. *Nutrition Journal* 7(15):1–8, 2007.

19. Davenport MH, Mottola MF, McManus R, Gratton R: A walking intervention improves capillary glucose control in women with gestational diabetes mellitus: a pilot study. *Appl Physiol Nutr Metab* 33(3):511–17, 2008.

20. Voldner N, Frøslie K, Bo KH, et al.: Modifiable determinants of fetal macrosomia: role of lifestyle-related factors. *Acta Obstet Gynecol Scand* 87:423–39, 2008.

21. Zimmerman FJ, Christakis DA: Children's television viewing and cognitive outcomes: a longitudinal analysis of national data. *Arch Pediatr Adolesc Med* 159(7):619–25, 2005.

22. Mendoza JA, Zimmerman FJ, Christakis DA: Television viewing, computer use, obesity, and adiposity in U.S. preschool children. *Int J Behav Nutr Phys Acta* 4:44, 2007.

23. Zimmerman FJ, Christakis DA, Meltzoff AN: Television and DVD/video viewing in children younger than 2 years. *Arch Pediatr Adolesc Med* 161(5):473–79, 2007.

24. Roberts DF, Foehr UG, Rideout V: Generation M: Media in the Lives of 8–18 Year-olds. Henry J. Kaiser Family Foundation, 2005. http://www.kff.org/entmedia/upload/Generation-M-Media-in-the-Lives-of-8-18-Year-olds-Report.pdf

25. Graves L, Stratton G, Ridgers N, Cable N: Comparison of energy expenditure in adolescents when playing new generation and sedentary computer games: cross sectional study. *BMJ* 335:1282–84, 2007.

26. Davis CL, Tomporowski PD, Boyle CA, et al.: Effects of aerobic exercise on overweight children's cognitive functioning: a randomized controlled trial. *Res Q Exerc Sport* 78(5):510–19, 2007.

27. Vehrs P: Strength training in children and teens: implementing safe, effective and fun programs. *ACSM's Health and Fitness Journal* 9(4):13–18, 2005.

28. American Academy of Pediatrics Committee on Sports Medicine and Fitness: Promotion of healthy weight-control practices in young athletes. *Pediatrics* 116 (6):1557–64, 2005.

29. Satter E: Children, the feeding relationship, and weight. *Md Med* 5(3):26–28, 2004.
30. Satter E: Feeding dynamics: helping children to eat well. *J Pediatr Health Care* 9(4):178–84, 1995.
31. Satter E: Eating competence: definition and evidence for the Satter Eating Competence model. *J Nutr Educ Behav* 39(5 Suppl):S142–53, 2007.
32. Fischer JO, Birch LL: Restricting access to palatable foods affects children's behavioral response, food selection and intake. *Am J Clin Nutr* 69(6): 1264–72, 1999.
33. Flynn M, McNeil D, Maloff B, et al.: Reducing obesity and related chronic disease risk in children and youth: a synthesis of evidence with 'best practice' recommendations. *Obes Rev* 7 (Suppl 1):7–66, 2006.
34. Saris W: Very-low-calorie diets and sustained weight loss. *Obes Res* 4:295s–301s, 2001.
35. Blair-West GW: Tantalus, restraint theory, and the low-sacrifice diet: the art of reverse abstraction: 10th International Congress on Obesity; September 4, 2006; Sydney, Australia - Symposium: obesity management: adding art to the science, invited presentation. *Med Gen Med* 9(4):18, 2007.
36. Jeffery R, Epstein L, Wilson G, Drewnowski A, Stunkard A, Wing R: Long-term maintenance of weight loss: current status. *Health Psychol* 19:5–16, 2000.
37. Theunissen MJ, Polet IA, Kroeze JH, Schifferstein HN: Taste adaptation during the eating of sweetened yogurt. *Appetite* 34(1):21–27, 2000.
38. Swithers S, Davidson T: A role for sweet taste: calorie predictive relations in energy regulation by rats. *Behav Neurosci* 122(1):161–73, 2008.
39. Dhingra R, Sullivan L, Jacques P, et al.: Soft drink consumption and risk of developing cardiometabolic risk factors and the metabolic syndrome in middle-aged adults in the community. *Circulation* 31(116):480–88, 2007.
40. Pereira M, Kartashov A, Ebbeling C, et al.: Fast-food habits, weight gain, and insulin resistance (the CARDIA study): 15-year prospective analysis. *Lancet* 365:36–42, 2005.
41. Hu F, Li T, Colditz G, Willett W, Manson J: Television watching and other sedentary behaviors in relation to risk of obesity and type 2 diabetes mellitus in women. *JAMA* 289:1785–91, 2003.
42. Manz F: Hydration in children. *J Am Coll Nutr* 26:562s–69s, 2007.
43. Committee on Nutrition: The use and misuse of fruit juice in pediatrics. *Pediatrics* 107(5):1210–13, 2001.
44. Schwartz M, Vartanian L, Wharton C, Brownell K: Examining the nutritional quality of breakfast cereals marketed to children. *J Am Diet Assoc* 108:702–705, 2008.
45. Fulkerson J, Story M, Neumark-Sztainer D, Rydell S: Family meals: perceptions of benefits and challenges among parents of 8- to 10-year-old children. *J Am Diet Assoc* 108:706–709, 2008.
46. Benton D: Role of parents in the determination of the food preferences of children and the development of obesity. *Int J Obes Relat Metab Disord* 28(7):858–69, 2004.
47. Dietz W, Birch L: *Eating Behaviors of the Young Child: Prenatal and Postnatal Influences for Healthy Eating*. Elk Grove Village, IL: American Academy of Pediatrics, 2008.

48. Mennella J, Jagnow C, Beauchamp G: Prenatal and postnatal flavor learning by human infants. *Pediatrics* 107:e88, 2001.

49. Forestell C, Mennella J: Early determinants of fruit and vegetable acceptance. *Pediatrics* 120:1247–54, 2007.

50. Satter E: *Your Child's Weight: Helping Without Harming (Birth Through Adolescence)*. Madison, WI: Kelcy Press, 2005.

51. Dreikurs R, Soltz V: *Children: The Challenge*. New York, Hawthorn Books, 1964.

52. Phelan TW: *1-2-3 Magic: Effective Discipline for Children 2–12*. 3rd ed. Glen Ellyn, IL: Parent Magic, 2003.

53. Olson R: Is it wise to restrict fat in the diets of children? *J Am Diet Assoc* 100:28–32, 2000.

54. Kranz S, Lin P, Wagstaff D: Children's dairy intake in the United States: too little, too fat? *J Pediatr* 151:642–46, 2007.

55. Rovner AJ, O'Brien KO: Hypovitaminosis D among healthy children in the United States: a review of the current evidence. *Arch Pediatr Adolesc Med* 162(6):513–19, 2008.

56. Cooke L, Wardle J, Gibson E, Sapochnik M, Sheiham A, Lawson M: Demographic, familial and trait predictors of fruit and vegetable consumption by pre-school children. *Public Health Nutr* 7:295–302, 2004.

57. Sullivan SA, Birch LL: Pass the sugar, pass the salt: experience dictates preference. *Dev Psychol* 26(4):546–51, 1990.

58. Leahy KE, Birch LL, Fisher JO, Rolls BJ: Reductions in entrée energy density increase children's vegetable intake and reduce energy intake. *Obesity (Silver Spring)* 16(7):1559–65, 2008

59. Desai BB: *Handbook of Nutrition and Diet*. Boca Raton, FL: CRC Press, 2000.

60. Batada A, Seitz M, Wootan M, Story M: Nine out of 10 food advertisements shown during Saturday morning children's television programming are for foods high in fat, sodium, or added sugars, or low in nutrients. *J Am Diet Assoc* 108:673–78, 2008.

61. Alvy LM, Calvert SL: Food marketing on popular children's web sites: a content analysis. *J Am Diet Assoc* 108(4):710–13, 2008.

62. Wang SY, Chen CT, Sciarappa W, Wang CY, Camp MJ: Fruit quality, antioxidant capacity, and flavonoid content of organically and conventionally grown blueberries. *J Agric Food Chem* 56(14):5788–94, 2008.

63. Asami DK, Hong YJ, Barrett DM, Mitchell AE: Comparison of the total phenolic and ascorbic acid content of freeze-dried and air-dried marionberry, strawberry, and corn grown using conventional, organic, and sustainable agricultural practices. *J Agric Food Chem* 51(5):1237–41, 2003.

64. Chassy AW, Bui L, Renaud EN, Van Horn M, Mitchell AE: Three-year comparison of the content of antioxidant microconstituents and several quality characteristics in organic and conventionally managed tomatoes and bell peppers. *J Agric Food Chem* 54(21):8244–52, 2006.

65. Butler G, Nielson J, et al.: Fatty acid and fat-soluble antioxidant concentrations in milk from high- and low-input conventional and organic systems: seasonal variation. *J Sci Food Agric* 88(8):1431–41, 2008.